Cancer
Prevention
and
Nutritional
Therapies

Other books by Richard Passwater include:

Trace Minerals, Hair Analysis and Nutrition (with Elmer Cranton, M.D.)
Chromium Picolinate
The Longevity Factor: Chromium Picolinate
The New Superantioxidant—Plus
SUPERNUTRITION: Megavitamin Revolution
SUPERNUTRITION for Healthy Hearts
Super Calorie, Carbohydrate Counter
The Easy No-Flab Diet
Selenium as Food and Medicine
The Slendernow Diet
Guide to Fluorescence Literature, Volumes 1-3

Cancer Prevention and Nutritional Therapies

Richard A. Passwater, Ph.D.

Keats Publishing, Inc.   New Canaan, Connecticut

Cancer Prevention and Nutritional Therapies is not intended as medical advice. Its intent is solely informational and educational. Please consult a health professional should the need for one be indicated.

CANCER PREVENTION AND NUTRITIONAL THERAPIES
Pivot Original Health Edition published in 1978 and a revised edition published in 1983 as *Cancer and Its Nutritional Therapies*.

Printed in the United States of America

Library of Congress Cataloging-in-Publication Data

Passwater, Richard A.
    [Totally revised and updated fact/book on cancer prevention and nutritional therapies]
    Cancer prevention and nutritional therapies,—Totally revised and updated ed.
      p. cm.
    Previous ed. published under title: Revised, updated fact/book on cancer and its nutritional therapies, 1983.
    Includes bibliographical references and index.
    ISBN 0-87983-607-5 (pbk.) : $14.95
    1. Cancer—Diet therapy. 2. Cancer—Nutritional aspects. 3. Cancer—Prevention. I. Title: Cancer prevention and nutritional therapies.
RC271.D52P37   1993
616.99′4—dc20   93-22989
                                                                                        CIP

Keats Publishing, Inc.
27 Pine Street, Box 876
New Canaan, CT 06840-0876

Contents

Cancer
Prevention
and
Nutritional
Therapies

CHAPTER 1

The Scope of This Book

Cancer Prevention and Nutritional Therapies will show you how to increase your protection against cancer so that you won't get cancer in the first place. This book will also help you overcome cancer if it is too late for protective measures. The information in earlier editions of this book has been proved by the test of time and the experience of thousands who have shared their success stories with me. *Cancer and Its Nutritional Therapies* was first published in 1978 and was updated in 1983. Those editions were based on my own research between 1968 and 1979, plus the research from a handful of other scientists. This is a complete revision that adds new information to the already proven information from the earlier editions.

Now leading scientists, including those of the National Cancer Institute (NCI), agree with the teachings of the earlier editions. I no longer have to rely primarily on my laboratory research and biochemical explanations—now I can also rely on the concurring findings of hundreds of studies of real people. These studies are so convincing that the NCI is funding dozens of large-scale clinical studies to provide the final data to conclusively prove the same conclusions I had come to through my earlier findings. I will discuss these findings in detail in later chapters.

You don't have to wait another twenty years for this final confirmation. The nutritional protective measures presented in this book are safe—and they will protect you not only against cancer but also against heart disease and many other diseases.

And I place my emphasis on YOU. You are the only person that can make the difference! It is up to you to protect yourself. You can choose to fight cancer before you get it or after you get it. You will not have to make drastic dietary changes. You can benefit from the protective measures presented in this book without changing your basic diet. However, those with bad diets will have additional benefit if they make at least some changes. This is a book that will help everyone, not just those who have "holier than thou" diets. I want to help real people in the real world. It does little good to preach dietary practices that people will choose not to follow. You can use the information in this book to select what protective modifications you can realistically make to your own lifestyle. It may be practical for you to merely add nutritional supplements to your diet now, and then when you are able, you may also make modifications such as to stop smoking or lower the fat content of your diet, if applicable.

The vast majority of cancers are preventable. Smoking and diet are responsible for most of these cancers. It goes without saying that because of the great risks of cancer and heart disease, no one should smoke. However, I understand that there are people, including my own family members, who have tried to stop smoking but have been unsuccessful so far. I encourage them to quit, but in the meantime, I want to protect them as much as possible. The evidence is that moderate smokers who are well nourished with antioxidant nutrients have less risk of cancer than nonsmokers who are poorly nourished.

I stated in *People* magazine in December 1980 that "No one under 80 should get heart disease and if you have enough vitamins and no genetic defects you can stop a cancer cell from ever forming." The guidelines in this book are a formula for a cancer-free life for millions of people. As I discussed in *The New Supernutrition,* "There is no such thing as a 100 percent guarantee of protection against cancer. Optimal nutrition will offer you greater protection against cancer than being undernourished." Several scientists have gone on record as to the involvement of diet as a cause of cancer, and their estimates range from 35 percent to 80 percent. However, these scientists have only considered the roles of the dietary factors such as fat and fiber that make up a large percentage of the diet, and they have overlooked much of the role of the micronutrients (vitamins and minerals) that protect against cancers caused by other agents such as smoking and chemicals in the environment. These cancers are not *caused* by poor diet, but micronutrients can stop their *promotion* into cancer. *This book details how to use micronutrients and reduction of exposure to cancer-initiating agents so as to achieve a 90 percent reduction in cancer risk and incidence!*

It's time for people to focus on the good news: not everything causes cancer, and easy lifestyle changes can protect against cancer. A few basic antioxidant nutrients—such as vitamin A and its precursor beta-carotene; vitamin C; vitamin E; and the trace mineral selenium—offer great protection against cancer. Hopefully, you will choose to eat more fruits and vegetables that contain these nutrients, but even if you don't, you can get these protective nutrients in many vitamin pills. Yes, you can protect yourself against many cancers by simply taking the right vitamins in the proper amount.

When Margaret Heckler was Secretary of the U.S. Department of Health and Human Services, she noted that 80 percent of all cancers in the U.S. were caused by smoking, what we eat and drink, too much sun exposure and other environmental factors. She said, "Too few realize the simple truth that cancer is often caused by the way we live, and its risks can be reduced by the daily choices we make in our lives. We know that the most important causes of cancer are the ones we can control. We are not always at the mercy of our environment. Environmental pollution accounts for only 2 percent of all cancer causes."

Dr. William DeWys of the NCI has estimated that diet causes about 35 percent of all cancers, tobacco causes about 30 percent, viruses about 5 percent, occupation about 4 percent, alcohol about 3 percent, excess sunshine about 3 percent, environmental pollution about 2 percent, medicine and medical procedures about 1 percent and food additives, 1 percent or less.

To fully understand how nutrients protect against cancer and help overcome it we must start with the basics. We will examine the question, "What is cancer?" If you don't really understand what cancer is, you probably won't be able to understand how cancer can be prevented or cured. Cancer is not just one disease or condition—it is a term used to describe over 100 diseases commonly known as "cancer." They are very similar, yet different enough to need slightly different approaches. Fortunately, the protective measures are nearly identical; it is the treatments that need to be individualized.

We continue to learn about cancer. We understand more about the roles of tumor initiators and promoters in the mechanisms of cancer formation. We are learning more about how cancers spread. This knowledge will lead to drugs that will actually halt these processes. However, we already know that certain nutrients prevent these processes, and we know how they prevent the initiation of cancer and help the immune system destroy existing cancers. We don't have to understand every last detail in order to take advantage of them.

Earlier, I mentioned that it is the treatments that have to be individualized. Let me be clear that nutritional therapy is compatible with any other therapy. *Cancer Prevention and Nutritional Therapies* is not intended to be used as a substitute for other therapies. I don't say that as a disclaimer to prevent me from being sued for practicing medicine. I am a research biochemist, not a physician, but the reason I make the statement is that my experience has been that it is better to take the best of both worlds than to use either one alone. Of course, there are good treatments and very bad treatments. I want to make the point right at the start that this book is intended to protect you from cancer via the intelligent use of nutrients, and to help you overcome cancer if you already have it. This book is not intended to encourage you to try to treat cancer with nutrition alone.

If you are wondering how nutrition can aid conventional chemotherapy, surgery and radiation techniques, it's by strengthening the immune system. The immune system is our last line of defense that can actually overcome existing cancer. But, this book will show you more than just how to revive and strengthen your immune system; it will show you how to protect yourself with earlier lines of defense against the factors that cause cancer.

In fact, our bodies are always at war with cancer. It's a constant battle and we have many defenses. My aim is to not only make you aware of how you can strengthen your existing defenses, but to show you how you can add to your armamentarium. This book will frequently discuss how to reduce the number of battles required, how to improve your personal defenses and how to help your body repair any damage that has already occurred.

The information presented in *Cancer Prevention and Nutritional Therapies* can help your body defend itself and even counterattack. Since the best defense is a good offense, you will learn how to activate your liver so that it can more effectively destroy invading chemicals that can cause cancer. You will also learn how to fortify your second line of defense—the membranes that are the skin of every cell, which keep cancer-causing agents from entering the cells. And even if these agents penetrate the cell, antioxidant nutrients will prevent the harmful reactions from occurring by destroying free radicals required to actually do the damage. These same nutrients aid the body in repairing damage and in strengthening the immune system, which can recognize and destroy cancer cells. We'll also look at how the "war on cancer" in general is going.

I'll get to the "how" to protect yourself and what to do if you have cancer later, but by now you are probably wondering a little about my experience with cancer research and why I am so sure that I can reduce your risk of cancer by 90 percent.

CHAPTER 2

My Research

My research led me to cancer research in 1970. Now I wasn't one of those scientists who instantly converted their research to cancer research because of the funds that were made available with President Nixon's "war on cancer." It seemed that, with the signing of the "Conquest of Cancer Act" in 1971, every scientist who was working in a related field all of a sudden redefined his or her research in terms of cancer to take advantage of the new funding source. Of course, it was the intent of the Act to draw more scientists into cancer research.

None of my research has ever been funded by the government, however. I announced my success in extending the lifespans of laboratory animals by using a combination of antioxidant nutrients at the 1970 annual meeting of the Gerontological Society in Toronto.[1] My research focused on stopping the deleterious effects in the body of very reactive chemicals called "free radicals." Today, the free-radical theory of aging is one of the most promising approaches to slowing the ravages of aging. In the 1960s there were very few of us working on this theory, which was developed by Dr. Denham Harman in the 1950s.[2] We will look at how free radicals cause cancer later.

At the gerontological meeting, another scientist wondered if my success in extending the lifespan of the laboratory animals could be due to a reduction in diseases such as cancer, rather than a slowing of the aging process. That comment struck a chord, as I could recall no apparent cancers in the antioxidant-protected animals, whereas the control groups receiving normal diets seemed to have occasional cancers.

When I returned to my laboratory, I designed a series of studies to determine if cancer prevention was a factor in the improved lifespans of the antioxidant-protected animals. As it turns out, the antioxidant nutrients protect against cancer and also protect against many secondary events that affect the lifespan. At this time, I still do not have evidence that the antioxidants affect the primary cause of aging, if there is one. However, now we know that free radicals are involved in over 60 human diseases, and that antioxidants can protect against the development of these diseases.

As I said, at this time there were few researchers looking at the detrimental role of free radicals in the body. Dr. Denham Harman of the University of Nebraska School of Medicine was investigating the roles of single nutrients on the lifespans of laboratory animals. Independently, Dr. Al Tappel of the University of California at Davis and I were studying combinations of antioxidant nutrients. Dr. Tappel was studying tissue levels of markers of free-radical damage such as lipofuscin, and I was studying actual longevity. Dr. Gerhard Schrauzer of the University of California at San Diego and Dr. Ray Shamberger of the Cleveland Clinic were studying a possible epidemiological link between selenium deficiency and cancer incidence. Dr. William Pryor of Louisiana State University and Dr. Lester Packer of the University of California at Berkeley were studying free-radical mechanisms. There were a few others close to this area of research, but this is the group that was progressing towards what now has been confirmed as the major link between diet and cancer.

In those days, to mention that cancer was linked to diet was blasphemous. To say that vitamins could protect against cancer was quackery. Of course, there are a few people around today who still are not convinced, but most scientists and physicians are aware of the evidence and now support the concept of protecting yourself from most cancers with antioxidant nutrients. Later, we discovered that these same nutrients stimulate the immune system to help the body overcome existing cancer in cases where the immune system hasn't been severely damaged by other treatments.

Also in those days, most research was directed towards proving how viruses caused cancer and developing vaccines to protect against cancer. With the war on cancer entrenching the leaders of the virus philosophy into leadership position in the new cancer bureaucracy, it was difficult to turn the research effort around from virus-vaccine to diet-prevention. It took two decades and many brave researchers who risked funding and peer acceptance to explore this new line of research.

In 1972, I filed for international patent protection for various combinations of nutrients that protected against cancer. These patents were granted in many countries, but in the U.S., it was like trying to patent a perpetual motion machine.[3] I also applied to the Food and Drug Administration for a new drug application to test the preventive powers of these antioxidant nutrients, but they denied permission because we couldn't agree on a protocol and they felt that these nutrients had not been proved safe.

In May 1973, I published "Cancer: New Directions" in *American Laboratory* and began a lecture series to challenge other researchers to join in the research.[4] Of course, at that time most scientists were skeptical, as they didn't know very much about this new concept of free-radical pathology. In fact, until *Prevention* magazine reported on my research in 1971, few people had even heard of free radicals.[5] Now free radicals and antioxidant nutrients are "buzz words" among the health minded. So I goaded skeptical scientists into trying to prove that I was wrong. Eventually, many laboratory animal studies were published confirming the protective role of antioxidant nutrients.

In 1975, I published the results of my cancer research in *Supernutrition: Megavitamin Revolution*.[6] By 1978, there was enough evidence based on animal studies to publish the first edition of *Cancer and Its Nutritional Therapies*.[7] At that time I cited hundreds of studies which showed that the deficiencies of certain vitamins and/or minerals increased the occurrence of both spontaneous and induced cancers. Conversely, many studies showed a dose-dependent relationship of nutrients to lowering the incidence of many cancers.

That is, the more of a nutrient that is consumed, the greater the reduction in cancer rates. This, too, was shown for spontaneous and induced cancers.

In 1978, I could also cite a few epidemiological studies showing that cancer incidence was inversely related to the amount of certain nutrients in the diet. Those who ate foods with low amounts of nutrients such as vitamins A, C or E, or the trace mineral selenium, had more cancers than those who ate more ample amounts.

On July 29, 1981, my research was presented to the National Cancer Institute (NCI). Attending the meeting were Dr. William Terry, Director of the NCI Division of Resources; Dr. John Mac-Donald, head of the NCI's Cancer Therapy Evaluation Program; Dr. Louis Carrese, Office of Program Planning and Analysis under NCI Director, Dr. Vincent DeVita; Dr. Richard Adamson, Director, Division of Cancer Cause and Prevention, NCI; Dr. Michael Sporn, Laboratory of Cancer Prevention; Dr. Mary Ann Sestili, Executive Secretary, NCI; Dr. Mitchel Heft, National Institute on Aging; Dr. Frank Rauscher, Vice President of Research, American Cancer Society; and others. They wanted more animal studies, more autopsies, and more development of the theory before they would agree to support my research.

Fortunately in 1981, there were a series of epidemiological studies published that confirmed the protective roles of these nutrients in real people, not just in laboratory animals. However, these epidemiologists lost sight of the laboratory animal research and thought that their research was standing alone. The two lines of research strengthen each other and my goal now is to show the epidemiologists the laboratory animal research and vice versa.

Maybe some good did come out of the presentation of my research to the NCI. By 1982, the NCI started a series of workshops to introduce the "free-radical cause of cancer" line of research to scientists and began funding small "pilot" studies. In June 1982, the National Academy of Sciences published a pamphlet entitled "Diet, Nutrition and Cancer." This booklet discussed the burgeoning line of evidence showing that certain nutrients could be protective, and that people should include more foods with fiber, vitamins A, C, E and the trace mineral selenium in their diets.

Fortunately, the strength of the research became sufficient to prod the NCI into funding dozens of large-scale clinical studies by the end of the 1980s to provide the conclusive evidence.

What is of interest to you is that my research has withstood the test of time and scrutiny of the scientific community. Also, what is of interest to you is that you do not have to rely on what I say, but as you will see throughout this book, you can rely on the evidence developed by hundreds of researchers who confirm what I say. And there are thousands of people out there who have told me how the information in the earlier editions helped them, and I am grateful for all of their "God Blesses." This is why I write this book. Please read it, check the research yourself, and discuss it with your health care provider. And may God bless you, too.

Now, let's check on the progress of the "war on cancer," and see what we can do about it.

REFERENCES

1. Plans for a large-scale study of possible retardation of the human aging process. 23rd Annual Meeting of the Gerontological Society, Toronto (October 21–24, 1970). Also see *Gerontologist* (1970) 10(3):11, 28.
2. The free-radical theory of aging. Harman, Denham. *Journal of Gerontology* (1956) 11:298–300.
3. US 39140 and others, US 97011 and others
4. Richard A. Passwater,"Cancer: New Directions," *American Laboratory* (1973) 5(6):10–22.
5. Don't age too fast. *Prevention* (Dec. 1971) 23(12):104–10.
6. Richard A. Passwater, *Supernutrition: Megavitamin revolution* (New York: Dial Press, 1975).
7. Richard A. Passwater, *Cancer and Its Nutritional Therapies.* (New Canaan, Conn.: Keats Publishing, Inc., 1978).

CHAPTER 3

Waging War on Cancer

The formal "War on Cancer" began with the National Cancer Act of 1971 passed by Congress and signed into law by President Richard Nixon on December 23, 1971. It was intended to be a "Christmas present" to the nation. The research community really didn't consider this the best approach, but the public and politicians felt better by throwing more money at the problem. The feats of the Manhattan Project and the Apollo Program were based on already existing scientific knowledge. The mechanisms of cancer are still not well understood.

Unfortunately, the additional money was not spent in new directions. It was channeled into more of the same research because those supporting the popular research at the time were promoted to direct this beefed-up program. Thus, they funneled the money into the same channels that got them to their respected positions.

The National Cancer Institute's (NCI) budget soared from $180 million in 1971 to $400 million in 1972. More than $22 billion and 20 years were spent before a new breed of scientists would convince the agency of the value of *prevention* via diet. So many people believed that with so many "promising" new drugs and treatments that a cure was in reach. A popular theme was "Cure cancer by America's 200th birthday in 1976."

Twenty years later, and with an annual NCI budget of more than $2 billion, more than 1.1 million Americans were diagnosed with cancer. One out of three living Americans could expect to

13

get cancer in his or her lifetime, and half of those who developed cancer that year would not survive five years. The *annual* death rate from cancer (in 1991: 514,000 Americans) is nearing the *total* deaths in battle from all U.S. wars (578,245).

Worldwide cancer rates are also increasing. About 2.3 million of the 11 million deaths that occur annually in industrialized nations are caused by cancer. When lung cancer is excluded, the cancer rate for men in industrialized nations has increased by 9 percent since 1950. Dr. Devra Davis of the National Academy of Sciences points out that the cancer rate is increasing above and beyond what we would expect due to aging or smoking.

In 1982, the war on cancer goal was changed to "a 50 percent reduction in cancer-related mortality on an age-adjusted basis by the year 2000." By 1982, the 20-year trend showed that the annual number of deaths due to cancer had *increased* by 55.7 percent. In 1962, 278,562 Americans died from cancer. In 1982, the number was 433,795. The incidence of cancer increased 25.1 percent, but after adjusting for age the increase was "only" 8.5 percent. The absolute cancer death rate per 100,000 persons increased 25.1 percent between 1962 and 1982, which when adjusted for age is 8.7 percent.

The researcher who published this comparison, Dr. John Bailar of the Harvard School of Public Health, concluded: "A shift in research emphasis, from research on treatment to research on prevention, seems necessary if substantial progress against cancer is to be forthcoming."[1] Just how to accomplish that goal is the subject of this book.

Later figures, comparing 1973 with 1987, show an age-adjusted *rise* in cancer incidence of 14.5 percent, with age-adjusted death rates increasing 5.4 percent. Much of that increase is attributed to smoking by women, as their lung cancer rate increased by 500 percent.

The death rate from cancer rose 0.2 percent from 1988 to 1989, while the death rate from heart disease fell 6 percent and the overall death rate fell 2.3 percent.

A report published by the American Hospital Association, "Meditrends 1991–1992," predicts that the number of people having cancer will double in the 1990s, making oncology instead of cardiology the leading specialty in the U.S. Cancer is already the

leading cause of death in women, but the report predicts that by
the year 2000, cancer will surpass heart disease as the leading cause
of death for everyone.

Dr. John Cairns, also of the Harvard School of Public Health,
stated in 1985 that there have been no significant gains in survival
from any of the major cancers since the 1950s. The so-called improvements in survival rates are merely artifacts of the increased
lead time due to earlier detection methods.

By 1991, the men's lung cancer rate was on the decline, but
aside from that there still wasn't much to brag about. The American Cancer Society had revised its estimate of a woman's lifetime
risk of breast cancer from one-in-ten to one-in-nine.

By 1991, the NCI had spent over a billion dollars on breast
cancer alone. According to NCI figures, 26.9 women out of every
100,000 died of breast cancer in 1973; by 1988, the number had
grown to 27.5 per 100,000. The Government Accounting Office
reported to Congress in 1991 that from 1976 to 1983, the five-
year survival rate for breast cancer increased 74 to 77 percent.
Importantly, changes in surgery and the management of the disease
have improved the quality of life for breast cancer patients.

Critics point to the large expenditures and insignificant progress.
They stress that new directions are needed. That was my theme
in 1973. NCI supporters counter the criticism—no matter what
year we are talking about—with glowing descriptions of how great
the latest developments just entering the experimental stages are.
It is unfortunate that they haven't panned out so far, but maybe
the next one will be significant. In the meantime, many cancer
researchers have discovered that great gains can be made in cancer
prevention with antioxidant nutrients. An ounce of prevention is
worth more than a pound of unsuccessful cure.

Ralph Moss, former public affairs director at Memorial Sloan-
Kettering Cancer Center in New York, writes in *The Cancer Industry* (New York: Paragon House, 1989):

"Our country is waging a billion-dollar war on cancer, and we seem
to be losing. . . . Conventional surgical, radiation and chemotherapy
treatments are often more devastating to the patient than the disease

itself . . . the cancer field continues to be marked by political power grabs and economic selfishness. With billions of dollars in research and treatment money . . . there is fierce competition. . . . Cancer patients seem to be the losers . . . while orthodoxy appears to have all the cards—money, power, prestigious credentials, influence in the major media—the continuing failure of orthodox medicine to deal satisfactorily with the major forms of cancer guarantees the growth of nonconventional approaches."

However, other scientists not involved in the "cancer industry" such as academic epidemiologists, are aware of the shortcomings of orthodoxy and they are also aware of the role of diet in preventing cancer. Several epidemiologists have become activists to bring the message of prevention to the establishment. I will report on their efforts in the chapters describing how nutrients protect against cancer.

Keep in mind that things often are the darkest just before the storm is over. There is good news to report on the rarer forms of cancer, for example. The five-year survival rate for children with leukemia has increased from 5 percent in the 1950s to 65 percent in 1981. Hodgkin's disease was almost always fatal before the 1960s and was almost always cured by the 1990s.

Survival rates have improved significantly for testicular cancer, bladder cancer, colorectal cancer, prostrate cancer and stomach cancer. Not all of the improvement is accounted for by increased lead time of early detection.

Lung cancer in men is on the decline. The other major cancers can be prevented as well by diet and lifestyle changes. It's up to you. Let's look at some of the lifestyle changes that can reduce your risk of cancer.

REFERENCES

1. John C. Bailar and Elaine M. Smith, "Progress Against Cancer?" *New England Journal of Medicine* (1986) 314:1226-32.

CHAPTER 4

Lifestyle Changes Prevent Most Cancers

I have already criticized the war on cancer for spending too much money on old ideas and not enough money on new directions for cancer research. A second major criticism is that not enough money is spent on educating the public about what they can easily do to reduce their risks. I am not advocating spending more money—just spending it in ways that result in saving more lives.

A group of 67 physicians and scientists under the auspices of Food and Water, Inc. held a news conference in February 1992 calling for Congress to insist that the National Cancer Institute spend more money on cancer prevention. Dr. Samuel Epstein of the University of Illinois said:

"Americans eat, breathe and work with cancer-causing substances because the government concentrates too much on diagnosing and treating the disease and not enough on preventing it. . . . The cancer establishment has minimized the evidence for increasing cancer rates which it has largely attributed to smoking and dietary fat, at the same time it has discounted or ignored the casual role of avoidable exposures to industrial carcinogens in the air, food, water and the workplace."

A year earlier, Dr. Epstein claimed that much of the money in the war on cancer

17

"has been squandered on a fruitless search for cancer 'cures.' Little has been done to prevent exposure to carcinogenic chemicals in the environment, despite ample evidence that chemical pollution of our air, water, food, and the workplace is the major cause of cancer. On the contrary, government, industry, and a small coterie of scientists have combined to stymie efforts to introduce preventive measures, such as strict pollution control standards. But cancer remains a preventable disease. It is up to citizens to push for action."[1]

OK, it seems that we have the "establishment" scientists with their opinion that we will soon have significant treatments and all we have to worry about is avoiding dietary fat, excess sunshine, and smoking. We have another, but smaller, group thinking that we spend too much effort on treatments and we have to worry more about pollutant chemicals. These two groups have been debating for years, but both should be paying more attention to our scientists who have a significant message about the role of antioxidant nutrients in preventing cancer. *Antioxidants protect against dietary fat, smoking, excess sun and chemical pollutants. They also improve response to other treatments by stimulating the immune response.*

Before we get into the new research that shows how antioxidant nutrients protect against cancer, let's review the ways in which all three groups agree that people can reduce their risks by simple lifestyle changes.

All three groups generally agree on the following, although there is debate on the amounts or degree:

1. Don't smoke or chew tobacco. Tobacco, alone or in combination with alcohol, remains the most important cause of cancer, accounting for about one in every three cancer cases occurring in the U.S. today. Limit exposure to secondhand smoke. (If you must smoke, antioxidants offer some protection.)
2. As far as dietary guidelines go, the key words are "moderation" and "fruits and vegetables." In general:
   • Maintain desirable body weight
   • Eat a varied diet

- Eat five servings daily of vegetables and fruits
- Eat foods rich in beta-carotene, vitamin A, vitamin C, vitamin E and selenium
- Eat ample amounts of fiber-containing foods such as whole-grain cereals, legumes, vegetables and fruits
- Reduce total dietary fat to 30 percent or less
- Limit alcohol consumption or don't drink alcohol at all
- Limit consumption of salt-cured, smoked or nitrate-preserved foods.

3. Limit exposure to sunlight.
4. Exercise or keep active.
5. Avoid heavy exposure to industrial and agricultural toxins.
6. Limit exposure to electromagnetic fields and X-rays.
7. Check your home radon level.
8. Get regular screening tests as advised for your age.

According to the establishment group, of each million new cancer cases, diet is related to about 350,000; tobacco causes about 300,000; viruses, about 50,000; occupational exposure to chemicals, about 40,000; alcohol, about 30,000; excess sunshine, about 30,000; environmental pollution, about 20,000; medicine and medical procedures, about 10,000; and food additives, 10,000 or less.

The second group feels that many more cancers are caused by various pollutants. Actually, when you consider that most Americans are not adequately protected by nutritional antioxidants, the true figure for "diet" is 700,000 to 800,000 or 70 to 80 percent. You don't have to worry so much about the "causes" if you are adequately protected with nutritional antioxidants. If you are genetically normal and follow the above advice, and optimally nourish yourself with the antioxidants, your total risk is decreased by 90 percent.

Now let's look at how the establishment applies this advice to each type of cancer. The following table shows the type of cancer and what the establishment believes is each type's major cause for a little over a million cancer cases in the U.S. in 1990.[2]

Cancer	Number	Percentage	Major Cause
Lung	157,000	16	tobacco
Colorectal	155,000	16	low-fiber, high-fat diet
Breast	150,900	15	ovarian hormones
Prostate	106,000	11	testosterone
Bladder	49,000	5	tobacco
Non-Hodgkin's lymphoma	35,600	4	(HIV, HTLV-1)
Uterine	33,000	3	estrogen
Oral & pharyngeal	30,500	3	tobacco, alcohol
Pancreatic	28,100	3	tobacco
Leukemia	27,800	3	X-rays
Melanoma	27,600	3	sunburn
Kidney	24,000	2	tobacco
Stomach	23,200	2	salt, tobacco
Ovarian	20,500	2	ovulation
Brain, nervous system	15,600	2	trauma, X-rays
Cervical	13,500	1	(papillomaviruses)
Liver	13,100	1	alcohol, hepatitis virus
Laryngeal	12,300	1	tobacco, alcohol
Thyroid	12,100	1	(iodine excess?)
Multiple myeloma	11,800	1	?
Esophageal	10,600	1	alcohol, tobacco

Even though there may be specific causes of these cancers, the antioxidant nutrients protect against cancer because they interfere with how the cancers form and stimulate the immune system to destroy any cancer cells that do develop.

Thus, it is incorrect to say that a deficiency of these nutrients "causes" cancer; rather, the deficiency allows the cancer to form when something else starts the process. Basically (up to a point) the more of the antioxidant nutrient that is present in your body, the less chance something has of starting a cancer. This has been proved in animal studies and confirmed by population studies.

In order to understand how the antioxidants prevent cancer, we need to know a little about the cancer process. You will see how cancers are started and how some agents—such as alcohol—promote the development of cancer.

REFERENCES

1. Samuel S. Epstein, "Losing the war against cancer: who's to blame and what to do about it," *Int. J. Health Serv.* (1990) 20(1):53–71.
2. Brian E. Henderson, Ronald K. Ross, and Malcom C. Pike, "Toward the primary prevention of cancer," *Science* (22 Nov. 1991) 254:1131–8.

CHAPTER 5

What Causes Cancer?

There is really no need to know how the antioxidant nutrients protect against cancer; all that we need to know is that they do. Studies have already established this as fact. This chapter is intended to help you understand cancer itself and how it develops. If you are just seeking practical how-to information on how to protect yourself against cancer, and you have no desire to understand more about cancer itself, then there is no need to read this chapter.

The National Cancer Institute (NCI) explains that cancer is really a group of diseases. There are more than 100 different types of cancer, but they all are a disease of some of the body's cells.

Most cancers involve tumors. The NCI explains tumor production as follows:

"Healthy cells that make up the body's tissues grow, divide, and replace themselves in an orderly way. This process keeps the body in good repair. Sometimes, however, normal cells lose their ability to limit and direct their growth. They divide too rapidly and grow without any order. Too much tissue is produced and tumors begin to form. Tumors can be either *benign* or *malignant*.

"Benign tumors are not cancerous. They do not spread to other parts of the body and they are seldom a threat to life. Often, benign tumors can be removed by surgery, and they are not likely to return.

"Malignant tumors are cancerous. They can invade and destroy nearby tissue and organs. Cancer cells also can spread, or metastasize, to other parts of the body, and form new tumors."[1]

The operative words are "unregulated growth of cells." What, then, causes cells to go astray? Whatever causes cell regulation to go astray is a cause of cancer.

Here are three common types of damage that alter the regulation mechanism of cells:

Membrane damage When a chemical reacts with components of the cell membrane—which is the "skin" of the cell—the sensors that tell the cell when to divide for growth can be damaged. If a sensor is damaged, then cell growth is uncontrolled; that is the *start* of cancer.

DNA damage If a chemical that enters the cell reacts with DNA—which is the "factory" of the cell that can reproduce cell components—the DNA can be damaged. If the DNA is damaged, it can make the wrong stuff or it can churn out more than is needed. If the wrong stuff is produced, then the cell becomes altered or "mutated." Mutated cells will grow quickly because they are not confined by quantities of similar cells. If the DNA churns out more cell material than needed, the cell is forced to divide and this results in uncontrolled tissue growth.

Immunosuppression Some chemicals, either directly or indirectly, inhibit the immune system from functioning properly. Although this is not direct damage to the cell's regulatory mechanism, it still involves part of the overall regulation of cell growth. One of the major roles of the immune system is to recognize mutated cells and destroy them. An impaired immune system may let mutated cells develop into cancers.

Cancer development is not a single-step process. We still need to learn much more about the multiple steps involved in the development of cancer. A third criticism of the war on cancer approach is that too much effort is devoted to random attempts to kill cancer cells with poisons, and not enough effort devoted to understanding the cancer development process.

In 1890, we had a better understanding of the tuberculosis process than we have in 1993 of the cancer process. Cancer is a complex, multi-step process in which cells accumulate multiple genetic alterations as they progress to a more malignant mutation. Nonetheless, we recognize three distinct phases of cancer development that we can halt with antioxidant nutrients.

One largely uncontrollable factor in cancer development is genetic susceptibility. Some of us have genes that cause cells to become mutated. These genes, called "oncogenes," often do not express themselves sufficiently to cause cancer until they become activated by certain agents including chemicals, radiation and viruses. Some cancers, such as small-cell lung cancer, may require as many as six independent oncogenes to trigger them.

Carcinogens Initiate Cancer

Here is how our 1993 knowledge shapes our thinking. People born with genetic abnormalities may have varying numbers of the required six oncogenes lying dormant and ready for activation. An analogy is an electronic device that operates by batteries. If six batteries are needed, the device won't operate until all six batteries are in place. The presence of the required oncogenes is like having the battery compartment loaded with fresh batteries. The device still will not operate, though, until the switch is activated. If all six oncogenes are inherited, they still won't start cancer development until all six oncogenes are activated by outside agents.

Others who inherit fewer oncogenes will not start the development process until sufficient normal genes are altered by some outside agent such as chemicals, radiation or viruses. In other words, the switch can be activated but unless the battery compartment is full, nothing will happen. Eventually, when all of the required oncogenes exist, then additional agents can activate them to start the cancer process.

Thus, some people may develop cancer very easily and others may never get cancer even though they are exposed to heavy amounts of cancer-causing substances. Consider the fact that not every smoker gets lung cancer and that some nonsmokers do. The genetically perfect individual who is well-nourished with antioxidant nutrients may never undergo enough genetic alterations to be able to switch on the cancer development process. On the other hand, a person who inherits all six oncogenes will only have to breathe relatively minor amounts of secondhand smoke or industrial fumes to activate the process.

Some cancers require little genetic alteration while others require much alteration. Similarly, some cancers require little activation and others require quite a bit of activation by the cancer initiation process.

The damage is caused by agents known as *carcinogens*. Carcinogens can damage critical parts of genes called proto-oncogenes, either directly or by generating free radicals. Carcinogens may be chemicals, radiation or viruses. Some chemicals considered to be carcinogenic actually do not cause cancer until the body converts them to another compound that is the true carcinogen. Sometimes other chemicals can convert a pre-carcinogen into a true carcinogen.

Your best protection is to not expose yourself to significant amounts of any carcinogen or pre-carcinogen. Since complete avoidance of carcinogens is not possible, try to limit your exposure and protect yourself with antioxidant nutrients. They will interfere with the mechanism that carcinogens use to do their damage, and they also interfere with many of the processes that convert pre-carcinogens into true carcinogens.

I described this process in my 1973 article, "Cancer: New Directions," and this knowledge is still state-of-the-art 20 years later.[2] It's just that now we have more convincing evidence to prove it.

Promotion

Keep in mind that initiating the development process does not necessarily lead to cancer. This process alone will only produce a series of independent precancerous cells. The process must be propagated to the point where these precancerous cells will reproduce, associate and develop their own blood supply and defense system. If there is no propagation or if the immune system is activated and destroys these precancerous cells, then there will be no cancer developed.

The next step in cancer development, called "promotion," allows the precancerous cells to reproduce rapidly and change their membrane surface properties to those characteristic of malignant cells. Anything that promotes cell reproduction decreases the chance that repair enzymes will repair (deactivate) the activated oncogene.

Compounds that increase cell reproduction (also called cell division, or mitosis) are commonly called "promoters." Cancer researchers call them "epigenetic carcinogens." Many promotors work by damaging growth suppressor genes or by inactivating components of the immune system. Common promoters include alcohol, hormones and polyunsaturated fats.

As an example, notice that smoking and drinking are co-carcinogens in esophageal cancer. Tobacco smoke components initiate the cancer by altering the DNA of the genes and then activating the altered genes. Alcohol becomes a factor because it promotes the development of cancer from the precancerous cells.

Studies have shown that even a single drinking binge can increase the cancer incidence. Rats injected with cancer cells and then given alcohol to the point of intoxication developed twice the number of tumors compared to those not receiving alcohol. Those who had blood levels of alcohol greater than 0.25 percent had eight times more tumors.[3]

It appears as if alcohol suppresses the ability of the immune system's "killer cells" to destroy cancer cells traveling in the bloodstream.

Progression

Even with promotion, the proliferating cells will not necessarily develop into cancer. The cell mass must grow large enough to affect body metabolism and start its own blood supply and defense system. This is where the immune system can do its job, unless it is impaired. Also, sometimes the altered cells are so defective that they just die off.

The multi-step cancer process can be summarized as follows:

1. Initiation
    a. Gene alteration
    b. Oncogene activation
2. Promotion
3. Progression
4. Cancer (carcinoma, adenocarcinoma)
5. Metastasis (spread to other areas)

It is important to note that antioxidant nutrients can protect against each and every step, although the same nutrients may not be protective against all steps. Some nutrients protect only at the initiation stage, some protect against promoters, and so on. A nutrient that is protective against one step may have no "special" use at later stages.

A specific antioxidant nutrient may protect by trapping free radicals to prevent the initiating damage, but if it works only to trap free radicals, then it will have no known value against existing tumors. Such a nutrient must be in the diet well in advance of developing full-scale cancer.

However, many free-radical trappers protect against several cancer development steps. As an example, vitamin E traps free radicals and it also works against existing cancers by stimulating the immune system. Even when the immune system doesn't completely overcome existing cancer on its own, a strong immune response often determines who is cured by a treatment and who isn't.

Hopefully by now you are curious about free radicals, free radical reactions and how antioxidant nutrients protect against them. This is explained in the next chapter.

REFERENCES

1. "What you need to know about cancer." *NIH Publication* 88–1566 (1988).
2. Richard A. Passwater, "Cancer: New directions." *American Laboratory* (1973) 5(6):10–22.
3. Gale Page, et al. (UCLA) Society for Neuroscience Annual Meeting, Anaheim (1992).

CHAPTER 6

The Battleground: Antioxidants Versus Free Radicals

If free radicals and antioxidants are just "buzz words" to you, this chapter may add to your understanding. However, it is not necessary to understand how antioxidant nutrients protect against cancer in order to take advantage of them. If you are interested, read this chapter, otherwise skip ahead to chapter seven.

My research has centered around free radicals and antioxidants for more than 30 years. It has always been result-oriented. I spend most of my time looking for better antioxidants and better ways for antioxidants to halt free radicals. The elucidation of the theory behind how antioxidants trap free radicals and how free radicals can cause the damage that can lead to cancer has been done by others such as Dr. William Pryor of the University of Louisiana and Dr. Lester Packer of the University of California at Berkeley.

Free Radicals

Let's start by defining a free radical. If this is the culprit we fear, then we should know something about it. A free radical is a very reactive chemical or chemical fragment. A free radical is defined as a compound or part of a compound that has an "unpaired" electron. The concept of an unpaired electron confuses many people who have had high school or college chemistry and are familiar with the charged chemical fragments called "ions."

A normal ion is a chemical fragment—either an atom, a molecule or a part thereof, that by losing or gaining one or more electrons has a net electrical charge. An isolated electron or positron can be considered an ion also, but let's keep things simple and ignore them for the purposes of this discussion. The charge of an ion can be either positive or negative. The strength of the positive charge depends on the number of missing electrons, and the strength of a negative charge depends on the number of extra electrons in the fragment. This has nothing to do with the directions of spin of the electrons.

In normal ions, the fragment always contains an even number of electrons, and these electrons are associated in pairs that spin in opposite directions. If somehow one of the electrons is removed from this normal arrangement, be it in a molecule or an ion, a nonpaired electron is left. This is a free radical.

Nature prefers molecules and ions to have paired electrons, as this is a lower energy state then when a nonpaired electron exists. When a free radical is created it usually doesn't last very long—normally a few millionths of a second. This is because it is not at the lower energy state that nature prefers. Therefore, the free radical tries to dissipate this extra energy and grab an electron from another molecule. That is where the damage occurs. By grabbing this electron from another molecule, another free radical is usually created. These reactions can go on and on in destructive chain reactions.

The resulting damage to cell components is much more severe than the damage one would think possible from one small initiating free radical. You can visualize this by considering the initial free radical as a nail in the road, and the resulting damage as many cars involved in a chain-reaction crash.

Some free radicals are not as dangerous as others. The harm done by free radicals depends on their number, where they are formed and the biological system involved.

Carcinogens readily produce free radicals and the body normally produces some free radicals. Oxygen can be made into a free radical called superoxide during normal metabolism. Superoxide is merely an oxygen molecule to which an electron has been added. This electron may be added in a variety of ways. A common way in which this may happen is when some reduced metal—such as iron or copper— might donate an electron to oxygen, thereby making superoxide.

Superoxide free radicals can be converted into a hydroperoxide. Hydroperoxides are not very reactive unless they are reduced by free iron or copper ions, in which case they are transformed into hydroxyl radicals. Hydroxyl radicals are quite reactive. They can be produced at an enormous rate and they persist sufficiently long to damage cellular proteins, fats and DNA. Fats are easy to damage by oxygen-radical attack. Fats can become free radicals called lipid peroxides which can, in turn, damage proteins. Hydroxyl radicals, which can be formed from oxygen during metabolism, can directly damage cellular proteins.

Free radicals can damage proteins in such a way that they are "cross-linked" together, which will impair their functional activity. Free radical cross-linking damage to DNA may impair its ability to open up to express genes. Enzyme function would also be impaired. The body has enzymes which can repair much of the damage to proteins, but when these enzymes become damaged themselves, repair processes are compromised.

If a large number of free radicals are produced by an acute exposure to carcinogens, then the body's antioxidant defense mechanisms may be overwhelmed. They will just simply not be able to cope with the load of free radicals, and this will initiate free radicals into crucial biological molecules, small molecules and macromolecules which can be propagated, leading to molecular damage, cross-linking and inactivation of functional activity.

Antioxidant Defenses

The body defends itself against minor numbers of free radicals with antioxidant nutrients and enzymes specifically designed to quench radicals. These substances include vitamin A, vitamin C, vitamin

E, coenzyme Q-10, beta-carotene and other carotenoids, the trace mineral selenium, and enzymes such as glutathione peroxidase, thiol enzymes, hydroperoxidases and superoxide dismutase (SOD).

The antioxidant nutrients quench free radicals by sacrificing themselves. This is what antioxidants do. Antioxidants are substances that react more easily with oxygen than the substances that they are intended to protect. In the process, the antioxidant nutrients become free radicals themselves.

One might ask, what does one gain by this? What one gains is that when the nutrients become free radicals, they are less reactive, longer-living radicals, and thus, not so dangerous to the biological system. Because they persist longer, the nutrient radicals can be converted back to their normal, protective, antioxidant forms. The net result is that the harmful free radicals have been destroyed and much of the antioxidant nutrients remain ready to protect again.

It has now been established that more than 60 human diseases involve free-radical damage, including cancer, heart disease and acceleration of the aging process. All that you really need to know is that your body is under constant free-radical attack, and that you need to keep your antioxidant defenses strong.

Carcinogens and pro-oxidants (such as fats and iron) increase the need for antioxidants. With that basic understanding, you are ready to look at the evidence that antioxidants protect against cancer.

CHAPTER 7

Vitamin A and Beta-Carotene

In the next several chapters I will present the evidence that antioxidant nutrients protect against cancer. I will also present some fundamental information about the amounts needed to achieve this protection. It may appear as if I am discussing them in alphabetical order, but that is a coincidence. Actually, I am discussing them in the order of their scientific interest.

This chapter will discuss vitamin A and its precursor, beta-carotene. Beta-carotene is still a strange sounding name to many people, but it is simply the name given to the compound that the body converts into vitamin A. Vitamin A is found in animal products such as liver, milk and eggs, whereas beta-carotene and other carotenoids are found in plant foods, primarily in yellow or orange vegetables, dark green leafy vegetables and some fruits.

Beta-Carotene and Other Carotenoids

People have always been told that carrots are good for your eyes because they are rich in vitamin A. In reality, carrots have no vitamin A! Carrots do have lots of beta-carotene and other carotenoids which are converted into vitamin A inside our bodies. The body has an enzyme that cleaves beta-carotene molecules in half to produce two vitamin A molecules.

"Big deal," you say, "the difference is only a technicality." Wrong! The difference is significant.

Beta-carotene and other carotenoids are nontoxic in the amounts that ordinarily can be consumed. Vitamin A, on the other hand, can be toxic in amounts that can be taken by the unaware. Another important difference is that the blood levels of the carotenoids are proportional to the dietary intake. By contrast, Vitamin A remains fairly constant over normal levels of intake, as "extra" amounts are removed from the blood and stored in the liver.

There is another distinction that may be important. Beta-carotene can neutralize "singlet oxygen," which can damage cells, and vitamin A cannot. There is evidence that beta-carotene can strengthen the immune function of cancer patients.[1]

Conversely, there are actions of vitamin A that beta-carotene does not have. Also, some people are not as efficient in converting beta-carotene and other carotenoids into vitamin A as they should be. Therefore, it is important to get both forms, vitamin A and carotenoids, in the diet for maximum protection.

Unfortunately, the U.S. Department of Agriculture surveys show that consumption of both vitamin A and carotenoids is below 70 percent of the RDA (recommended dietary allowance, which doesn't even consider the extra need for cancer prevention) for 31 percent of Americans, and below 60 percent of the RDA for 23 percent of Americans.[2,3] Typical American diets contain about 1.5 milligrams of beta-carotene daily. They should contain at least 5 to 6 milligrams daily, and be supplemented with 15 to 25 milligrams daily.

Beta-carotene is the best protector against cancer of the 20-some carotenoids normally found in food. The next best are alpha-carotene, lycopene, lutein and canthaxanthin. All of these carotenoids, with the exception of lycopene, can be converted into vitamin A in the body.

There will always be some who contend that we still don't know if it is the vitamin A or carotenoids that are protective, or other factors in fruits and vegetables that are the true protective factors. There is no question that vitamin A and carotenoids themselves protect against cancer. This has been demonstrated in laboratory animal tests in which vitamin A and/or carotenoids alone have shown a dose-related protection against cancer. I have shown that vitamin A and other antioxidant nutrients, alone, have reduced cancer incidence by over 90 percent. However, a study designed to elucidate the answer to the question was published in 1991. It concluded that "the (main) cancer-protective factor is carotene, rather than another component or combination of components of vegetables and fruits."[4]

Do not interpret this conclusion as saying that fruits and vegetables have no other cancer-preventing values. They contain many nutrients and other compounds, including fiber and enzyme promoters, that offer some protection against cancer. The point is, vitamin A and carotenoids themselves do protect against cancer, and you should take advantage of them. Eat your fruits and vegetables but also supplement your diet with appropriate amounts of vitamin A and carotenoids as discussed at the end of this chapter.

Vitamin A's Protective Action

I will discuss vitamin A and beta-carotene first for two reasons; first, vitamin A has been associated with cancer prevention longer than any other nutrient, and second, because vitamin A is involved with cancer prevention in three ways.

The evidence that vitamin A was protective against cancer first came to light shortly after its discovery in 1913 by McCollum and Davis.[5] In the early 1920s two reports associated vitamin A deficiency with cancer-like changes in mucous tissue cells lining the trachea, larynx and bronchi.[6,7] Several studies from the 1930s through the 1950s confirmed that vitamin A functions in the maintenance of normal tissue and control of cellular growth, and that deficiency produces metaplastic changes.

By the mid-1950s studies were showing that vitamin A regulates the series of events in the development of the differences in types of cells. Thus, the first way in which vitamin A (not the carotenoids) is involved in cancer prevention is through regulation of cell growth and development. This is greatly different from the second way (for both vitamin A and carotenoids), which is antioxidant protection against free radicals. A third way is that the carotenoids and vitamin A both enhance the communication between cells so that mutated cells cannot cause other mutated cells to grow. This line of research examines the relationship between carotenoids and synthesis of a "gap-junction" protein called *connexin*.[8] Cells can communicate with other cells either by having a cell secrete growth factors that travel to another cell, or by direct contact with information exchanged across gap junctions.

The regulation of growth and differentiation is also important in helping to return cancerous cells back to normal. As I reported in the early editions of this book, as early as 1974 researchers were aware of the potential of vitamin A.

Dr. Frank Chytill of Vanderbilt University was quoted as saying, "Recent dramatic findings about vitamin A and its effects on cancer have opened up a whole new approach to cancer therapy." Dr. George Plotkin of the Massachusetts Institute of Technology was quoted as saying that "Vitamin A deficiency doesn't cause cancer, but it makes the body less able to resist cancer." He found that giving rats ten times their usual vitamin A intake dramatically slashed their susceptibility to lung cancer.

Now this was no longer involving vitamin A deficiency. The researchers now were crossing over into the protective role of extra amounts of vitamin A, as I had found in 1972.[9]

In 1975, Norwegian researcher Dr. E. Bjelke did a study of 8,278 men and found that carotenoids protected against lung cancer. (Vitamin A itself was not studied.)[10] However, few researchers paid any attention to these findings.

In a December 1977 discussion I had with Dr. Michael Sporn at the National Cancer Institute (NCI) he stressed:

"If you are vitamin A-deficient, there is no question that you may be more susceptible to development of cancer. . . . Probably one of your best investments that you can make in your food budget is to spend a few cents a day and take a multivitamin capsule.

"Well over half of all human cancer starts in epithelial tissue: the tissue that forms the lining of organs, forms glands such as mammary glands, skin, and passages in the body. The respiratory tract, the digestive tract, the urinary tract, and the reproductive tract are all lined with epithelial tissue. And all of the specialized cells that form epithelial tissue depend on vitamin A for their normal development.

"Vitamin A is a hormone-like controller of cell differentiation. The approach that we are trying to develop is to use vitamin A derivatives, not to kill cancer cells, but to control the differentiation of precancerous cells."

What Dr. Sporn meant by "controlling cell differentiation" is to keep the cells in a mature differentiated state, rather than reverting back to the undifferentiated cells that are characteristic of cancer.

Dr. Sporn is an NCI pioneer in prevention of cancer. This approach was almost unheard of in the mid-1970s. Dr. Sporn explains:

"If all you do is just slow down this process of development of cancer so that instead of the typical twenty-year latent period from the time people may be first exposed to a carcinogen and the time that they develop cancer, you double the latent period, then there would be twenty additional years of good life that you would be offering people.

"Now in terms of modern surgery and chemotherapy, if they get an additional five years of survival, this is considered a very major achievement. So what we are really trying to do is to slow down or prevent the development of malignancy.

"If you slow it down enough, then for practical purposes it never occurs, although the basic process of development of cancer may still be going on, but at a very, very slow rate—such that it really never causes anyone any problems.

"The latent period is like a fire that is smoldering beneath the surface. It gives no symptoms; but if one goes and looks for precancerous cells, you can find evidence of the chronic disease process. The object of the preventive approach as I see it is to do something about the disease process when it is in the early, smoldering stage, before you have the fire. Once you have invasive cancer, then you can't do prevention anymore. You have to change your approach.

"It's pretty clear that vitamin A has hormone-like action in controlling cell differentiation. Cancer would appear to be a disease in which the gene material, DNA, has been damaged by chemicals or radiation. Usually, the damage will kill the cells, but sometimes the damage leads to cancer.

"Once DNA is damaged, cancer doesn't occur immediately. It can be twenty years after DNA damage occurs before malignancy develops."

Conclusive Scientific Evidence

In 1979, a study of 25,000 Japanese showed that beta-carotene protected against cancers of the lung, stomach, colon, prostate and cervix.[11]

However, in spite of the many animal studies, the few epidemiological studies, my lectures, articles and book on the subject, and the pioneering interest of Dr. Sporn at NCI, the role of nutrition in preventing cancer did not arouse a lot of interest. It wasn't until internationally famous researchers in the cholesterol field "discovered" the role of vitamin A in preventing cancer in 1981. Their reputations drew interest to the field. Who cares who gets the credit as long as the information gets disseminated so that the public can benefit?

The landmark paper was published by Dr. Jeremiah Stamler of Northwestern University School of Medicine and various colleagues at three other institutions.[12] This study followed 1,954 middle-aged men for 19 years. It compared the incidence of cancer in four groups, depending on how much vitamin A and carotenoids they had in their diet.

Men in the lowest quartile of vitamin A intake had seven times the incidence of lung cancer compared with those in the top quartile. For 30-year smokers, the protection of vitamin A was even greater—those in the lowest quartile had 8.1 times as much lung cancer as those in the top quartile of vitamin A intake. The following table summarizes the findings:

Vitamin A Intake Quartile	Relative Lung Cancer Risk	
	All Men	Smokers
lowest	7.0	8.1
2nd	5.5	5.6
3rd	3.0	3.9
highest	1.0	1.0

Table 7.1 shows the three-dimensional graph of the results, plotting vitamin A intake against duration of smoking and the incidence of lung cancer. Note that nonsmokers consuming the most vitamin A had no lung cancers. Also note that moderate smokers consuming more vitamin A had fewer lung cancers than non-smokers receiving little vitamin A.

In 1982, the Committee on Diet, Nutrition and Cancer of the National Research Council, National Academy of Sciences published its report, "Diet, Nutrition and Cancer."[13] It concluded, "Epidemiological evidence is sufficient to suggest that foods rich in carotene or vitamin A are associated with a reduced risk of cancer."

Now the floodgates of research were opened. Many researchers took note and began publishing scores and scores of research studies.

The picture is clear to most scientists working in the field: Vitamin A and carotenoids protect against many types of cancer. Many scientists are calling for the Food and Drug Administration (FDA) and the Life Sciences Research Office of the Federation of American Societies for Experimental Biology (FASEB) to look at many new studies and to re-examine their positions.

However, unequivocal scientific proof awaits prospective clinical trials in humans. It is doubtful if official agencies will recommend supplements of vitamin A and beta-carotene until the final evidence is in. These studies are under way, and the results should start coming in by the late 1990s. In the meantime, I advise you to consider fortifying your diet with appropriate amounts of vitamin A and carotenoids. Remember the recommendations by the NCI and the American Cancer Society to eat more foods rich in vitamin A and beta-carotene.

Prevention

Dietary recommendations for vitamin A and carotenoids for reducing your risk of cancer are as follows:

1. Eat a varied diet that includes five daily servings of fruits and vegetables.
2. To ensure adequate carotenoid and vitamin A levels, consider taking a daily vitamin supplement containing the following: 5,000 to 10,000 IU of vitamin A, 15 to 25 milligrams of beta-carotene (25,000–42,000 IU). Formulas containing other carotenoids may become available in the future.

Therapy

Vitamin A and the carotenoids can help any proven therapy known at this writing, because they stimulate the immune system and help cells mature into normal cells. Although several of the unproven dietary cancer therapies stress fruits and vegetables and their juices that are rich in the carotenoids, I have no scientific basis for recommending such approaches alone. My emphasis is to use these nutrients along with conventional therapies.

The levels of vitamin A and carotenoids listed for prevention should also serve well for adjunct therapy, unless directed otherwise by your health care professional.

REFERENCES

1. George S. Hughes, "The effects of beta-carotene on the immune system in cancer," Nutr. Rep. (1992) 10(1):1–8.

2. E. M. Pao and S. J. Mickle, "Problem nutrients in the United States," *Food Techn.* (1981) 35:58–79.

3. A. F. Grocetti and H. A. Guthrie, "Nutrient quality of diets of respondents from nationwide food consumption survey, 1977–78," USDA Conference, Washington, D.C., (Nov. 1982).

4. R. Harris, et al., "A case-controlled study of dietary carotene in men with lung cancer and in men with other epithelial cancers," *Nutrition and Cancer* (1991) 15:63–8.

5. E. V. McCollum and M. Davis, "The necessity of certain lipids in the diet during growth," *Journal of Biological Chemistry* (1913) 15:167–75.

6. S. Mori, "The changes in the para-ocular glands (in vitamin A deficient diets)," *Johns Hopkins Bulletin* (1922) 33:357–9.

7. S. B. Wolbach and P. R. Howe, "Tissue changes following deprivation of fat-soluble A vitamin," *Journal of Experimental Medicine* (1925) 42:753-77.

8. George Wolf, "Retinoids and carotenoids as inhibitors of carcinogenesis and inducers of cell-cell communication," *Nutrition Reviews* (1992) 50(9):270–4.

9. Patent application US 39140, US 97011 and others.

10. E. Bjelke, "Dietary vitamin A and lung cancer," *International Journal of Cancer* (1975) 15:561–5.

11. T. Hirayama, "Diet and cancer," *Nutr. Cancer* (1979) 1:67–81.

12. Richard B. Shekelle et al., "Dietary vitamin A and risk of cancer in the Western Electric Study," *Lancet* (Nov. 28, 1981) 2:1185–90.

13. Committee on Diet, Nutrition and Cancer, National Academy of Sciences, *Diet, Nutrition and Cancer* (Washington, D.C.: National Academy Press, 1982).

CHAPTER 8

Vitamin C Against Cancer

In the summer of 1990, I had difficulty believing that what I was hearing was true. The National Cancer Institute was cosponsoring a symposium to examine the biologic functions of vitamin C *and its possible relation to cancer.* Scientists at the NCI's Division of Cancer Prevention and Control were so impressed by the over one-hundred epidemiological studies showing that vitamin C protected against cancer that they invited over 130 scientists from around the world to discuss the topic September 10th through the 12th, in 1990. They even invited Dr. Linus Pauling, after years of discounting his work. The two-time Nobel Laureate had the last laugh.

One summary of this historic conference stated, "Evidence continues to accumulate that vitamin C has numerous biologic effects, including some that may relate to the prevention of cancer."[1] Another summary noted that "the data caused many participants to reconsider the importance of this agent in physiologic and clinical events."[2]

At this landmark conference, the action of vitamin C against free radicals was discussed, along with the way in which this action prevents cancer. Several studies described the role of vitamin C in immune function. Vitamin C can concentrate in neutrophils and lymphocytes to supercharge them against viruses, bacteria and damaged cells.

Researchers reviewed many of the laboratory animal studies that

42

showed vitamin C reduced cancer incidence. Out of the 75 epidemiological studies that were reviewed, 54 unequivocally demonstrated "significant evidence of a reduced risk for cancers in persons with a higher intake of vitamin C."[3]

Conference members even discussed the "several studies [which] found that vitamin C enhanced the effectiveness or reduced the toxicity of traditional cancer therapies."[2] Well, these findings have been my theme since 1973, and are the subject of this book.

Later, newspaper headlines informed us that high vitamin C intake resulted in longer life.[4] It is so exciting to see the NCI finally funding studies on vitamin C and cancer. When I first wrote *Cancer and Its Nutritional Therapies,* absolutely no funds were being spent in this area. Even Dr. Linus Pauling, who had presented data in 1976 that vitamin C benefited cancer patients, couldn't get funding.[5] Anyone who wanted to investigate this area either had to use their personal funds or bootleg the research with funds from other projects.

Even before the NCI conference on vitamin C, the U.S. Surgeon General concluded that human studies did show a protective association between foods containing vitamin C and cancers of the esophagus, stomach and cervix.[6] The National Research Council's "Diet and Health Report" concluded that epidemiological studies did suggest that vitamin C-containing foods such as citrus fruits and vegetables may offer protection against cancer.[7]

In February 1992, Dr. Gladys Block (who had relocated from the NCI to the University of California at Berkeley) called upon other scientists to petition the Food and Drug Administration (FDA) to consider allowing the information about vitamin C's protective action against heart disease to be given the status of an official health claim. She pointed out that although every study was not the ultimate in scientific design (none are), the preponderance of evidence suggested that vitamin C and the other antioxidant nutrients are protective against cancer.

Dr. Block stated in her letter to other scientists that:

"I have reviewed the epidemiologic literature, about 140 studies, on the relationship between antioxidant micronutrients or their food sources and cancer risk. The data are overwhelmingly consistent. With possibly fewer than five exceptions, every single study is in the protective direction, and something like 110 to 120 studies found *statistically significant* reduced risk with high intake."

The Roles of Vitamin C Against Cancer

I have already discussed the role of vitamin C as an antioxidant nutrient that traps free radicals. It does more than that. Not only are the reactions that vitamin C is *directly* involved in important, but the reactions that vitamin C is *indirectly* involved in as well. Recently we have begun to understand two additional functions of vitamin C. These functions were reviewed by Dr. Harish Padh of the University of Chicago.[8]

The first new realization involves vitamin C's role as an antioxidant. Not only is vitamin C an antioxidant in terms of protecting body components by scavenging free radicals, but vitamin C is an antioxidant in the sense that it keeps the mineral portions of certain enzymes in their proper reduced electronic state.

Minerals such as iron and copper are key components of hundreds of enzymes. This includes copper in monooxygenases and iron in dioxygenases. Enzymes control body chemistry. Nearly every type of reaction in the body requires a specific enzyme. Enzymes that depend on iron and copper won't work if these minerals are oxidized to a higher electronic valance state. Vitamin C restores this required electronic state and thus rejuvenates oxidized enzymes.

Dr. Padh concludes, "The available data suggest that perhaps the most significant role of ascorbate is as a reductant that, along with other reducing agents, minimizes damage by oxidative processes. This role includes keeping iron and copper ions in some enzymes in their required reduced form and neutralizing harmful oxidants and free radicals."

When you add to this the new comprehension that cells can hold and use more vitamin C than previously thought, all of a sudden we can begin to explain how megavitamin or orthomolecular levels of vitamin C work.

The concentration of ascorbic acid in cells could be as high as several millimoles, considerably higher than previous estimates. This applies to human peripheral mononuclear leukocytes, which include monocytes, B lymphocytes, and T lymphocytes (T-cells).

The report also remarks, "The new data come after learning that neutrophils appear to have both low-affinity and high-affinity membrane transporters for ascorbic acid. . . . having two transport systems of different affinities and capacities gives cells the flexibility to respond and adjust to quite different extracellular concentrations of the vitamin."

Now we know that cells of the immune system can hold considerably more vitamin C than once believed. In addition, we now learn that cells have two mechanisms of vitamin C uptake. There must be a reason!

In addition, vitamin C regenerates vitamin E, which is also an antioxidant nutrient. Vitamin C prevents dietary nitrates and nitrites from being converted into cancer-causing nitrosamines. But, perhaps most importantly, vitamin C enhances the immune system.

In my earlier books, I discussed the research of NCI researchers Drs. Paul Chretien, T. F. Fehniger and Robert Yonomoto, who showed that 5 grams of vitamin C daily increased the production of lymphocytes (white blood cells without granules) when the body was threatened by foreign substances, and that 10 grams daily produced an even greater effect.[9]

As long ago as 1971, the importance of vitamin C to the immune system was known. Drs. Lawrence DeChatelet, Charles McCall and Robert Cooper reported vitamin C stimulated increased activity of white blood cells. Without copious amounts of vitamin C, white cells can engulf bacteria, but they cannot break down the bacteria.

Cancer patients have a poor ability to make new lymphocytes, and their ability to survive is in line with their ability to produce lymphocytes. After surgery, radiation treatment and most chemotherapy, the immune system is very weak. Even marginal vitamin C deficiency affects immunity, as demonstrated by researchers at the UCLA School of Public Health in Los Angeles.[10] This is why I strongly recommend nutritional therapy as an adjunct to conventional cancer treatments, unless specially contraindicated by the attending physician.

Cancer Therapy

Of course I am not the only one who advocates using vitamin C along with other treatments for cancer. The study I referred to earlier by Dr. Pauling was begun in 1971 with the help of Dr. Ewan Cameron of Vale of Leven Hospital, Loch Lomondside, Scotland. The Cameron and Pauling study compared the results for 100 terminally ill cancer patients given 10 grams (10,000 milligrams) of vitamin C daily to the results for 1,000 cancer patients treated by conventional therapy without using adjunct vitamin C. Both groups of patients were treated by the same physicians in the same hospital.

At the time the study report was prepared, those patients given vitamin C had lived more than four times longer than the matched "control" patients. When I wrote *Cancer and Its Nutritional Therapies* in 1978, 13 of the vitamin C patients were still alive, with 12 of them apparently free of cancer. At that time, the survival ratio was more than five times longer for the vitamin C group, and still improving. All of the 1,000 "control" patients had died.

Sixteen of the 100 vitamin C supplemented patients lived more than a year, as opposed to only three of the 1,000 patients not given vitamin C.

The patients selected for this vitamin C trial had been pronounced terminal. In the considered opinion of at least two independent physicians, the continuance of any conventional form of treatment would offer no further benefit.

At the time of the 1976 report, 13 vitamin C-treated colon cancer patients had lived more than seven times as long as the 130 matched control patients. And their quality of life improved and pain lessened. The 1976 report also indicated that the vitamin C-treated breast cancer patients lived six times longer than their matched control group, and vitamin C-treated kidney cancer patients lived five times longer.

Drs. Cameron and Pauling also noted that survival time was increased by a factor of at least twenty for some 10 percent of the patients. This caused them to wonder what the results would be if treatment were started earlier and if larger amounts of vitamin C were used.

Dr. Pauling recommends that if we are apparently healthy that we get at least 18 grams (18,000 milligrams) of vitamin C daily for optimal nourishment. Sick people need more, depending on their disease and its severity. Cancer patients should consult Dr. Pauling's books *Cancer and Vitamin C* and *How to Live Longer and Feel Better*.[11,12]

At this writing Dr. Pauling is conducting a follow-up study with Dr. Abram Hoffer of Victoria, British Columbia, Canada. The study came about serendipitously. Oncologists were referring cancer patients to Dr. Hoffer, a psychiatrist, for treatment of their depression and anxiety. His treatment of the symptoms included antioxidant nutrients. He noticed that the patients on the nutritional therapy were doing better than normally expected.

Drs. Hoffer and Pauling combined their efforts to study 134 cancer patients referred to them between April 1988 and April 1989. Normally, terminally ill cancer patients such as those referred to Dr. Hoffer would be expected to live an average of five to six months. However, most of those who were given the nutritional adjunct therapy were still alive in late 1992. Dr. Pauling notes that they are living an average of 15 times longer than would otherwise be expected, given their cancers.

The fact that vitamin C extends the lives of cancer patients was confirmed by Drs. Akira Murata and Fukumi Morishige of Saga University in Japan in 1981.[13] In their study, patients who received 5 to 30 grams of vitamin C daily as their only therapy lived an average of 6.2 times as long as those on a dosage of 4 grams of vitamin C or less per day. Those suffering from cancer of the uterus who took vitamin C lived an average of 15.4 times longer than those receiving little or no vitamin C supplementation.

In 1985, Dr. Morishige and his colleagues improved their cancer treatment by adding a copper compound with the vitamin C therapy. This treatment has been very effective in animal studies and with human cancer patients.[14]

The Cameron and Pauling study was published in 1976, but the orthodoxy did not believe a vitamin could be involved in preventing or healing cancer at that time. Unfortunately, the only physicians who utilized this adjunct therapy were the holistic physicians who regularly incorporate nutritional advances into their practices in spite of censure and harassment by the orthodoxy. The holistic physicians testify that they are getting better survival rates and better quality of life for their patients using the antioxidant nutrients, especially vitamin C.

Unfortunately, the orthodox not only did not welcome the advancements made by Dr. Pauling's research, they attempted to destroy it. A study made at the Mayo Clinic was widely purported to show that vitamin C did not work; however, the study was completely inadequate.[15] In the Mayo Clinic study, vitamin C was given to patients for only 10 weeks, and not continually for the rest of their lives, as was the protocol in the Cameron and Pauling study. None of the Mayo Clinic patients died while receiving vitamin C. Their deaths occurred only after vitamin C had been discontinued.

Prevention and Therapy

As I mentioned earlier, Dr. Pauling suggests that even healthy persons should get 18 grams of vitamin C daily. The RDA is only 60 milligrams, but this RDA does not consider the role of vitamin C in protecting against cancer, heart disease and other diseases beyond the deficiency disease, scurvy.

I would suggest that you consider at least 2 to 4 grams daily for prevention, if you choose not to follow the excellent advice of Dr. Pauling for some reason. For therapy, I suggest you read Dr. Pauling's books mentioned earlier.

There are less acidic forms of vitamin C available such as mineral ascorbates, which are easier on the digestive system than the ascorbic acid form of vitamin C.

There is also a new development to consider. A new form of vitamin C appears to be better absorbed and is available to the body longer, according to preliminary research. This form of vitamin C includes a vitamin C metabolite called L-threonic acid or calcium threonate.

In 1991 *The FASEB Journal,* the official journal of the Federation of American Societies for Experimental Biology, reported two studies shedding more light on the role of the vitamin C metabolite, L-threonic acid. The first study showed that this vitamin C metabolite increases the amount of vitamin C taken up by T-cells of the immune system.[16] The second study showed that this metabolite increases the action or "potency" of vitamin C.[17] The vitamin C metabolite, L-threonic acid, is available as a food supplement only in the patented vitamin C formulation having the trademark Ester-C.

In June 1992, a more detailed report of the role of this metabolite in potentiating the action of vitamin C in preventing scurvy was published in *Life Sciences.*[18]

REFERENCES

1. Donald Earl Henson, Gladys Block, and Mark Levine, "Ascorbic Acid: Biologic functions and relation to cancer," *Journal of the National Cancer Institute* (April 17, 1991) 83(8):547-50.
2. Gladys Block, Donald Earl Henson, and Mark Levine, "Vitamin C: A new look," *Annals of Internal Medicine* (1991) 114(10):909-10.
3. Gladys Block, "Vitamin C and cancer prevention: The epidemiological evidence," *American Journal of Clinical Nutrition* (1991) 53:270S-282S.
4. Susan FitzGerald, "Take your vitamins—and you may live longer," *Philadelphia Inquirer* (May 8, 1992) 325(128):1,A16.
5. Linus Pauling and Ewan Cameron, *Proceedings of the National Academy of Sciences* (Oct. 1976) 73(10):3685-9.
6. U.S. Department of Health and Human Services, *The Surgeon General's report on nutrition and health* (Washington, D.C.: U.S. Government Printing Office, 1988).

7. Committee on Diet, Nutrition, and Cancer, National Research Council, *Cancer, Diet and Health: Implications for reducing chronic risk* (Washington, D.C.: National Academy Press, 1989) p. 593–605.

8. Harish Padh, "Vitamin C: Newer insights into its biochemical functions," *Nutrition Reviews* (Mar. 1991) 49:3 65–70.

9. Robert H. Yonomoto, Paul B. Chretien, and T. F. Fehniger, "Ascorbic acid enhances lymphocyte production." *Proceedings of the American Society of Clinical Oncology* (1976) 288.

10. R. Jacob, "Immunocompetence and oxidant defense during ascorbate depletion in healthy men," *American Journal of Clinical Nutrition* (1991) 54:1302S–1309S.

11. Ewan Cameron and Linus Pauling, *Cancer and Vitamin C* (NY: Warner Books, 1981).

12. Linus Pauling, *How to Live Longer and Feel Better* (NY: Freeman and Co., 1986).

13. Akira Murata and Fukumi Morishige, International Conference on Nutrition, Tianjin, China (June 1981) (Reported in *Medical Tribune* July 22, 1981).

14. Lewis Vaughn, "Vitamins against cancer: News from the front," *Prevention* (June 1985) 28–30.

15. E. T. Creagan, et al., "Failure of high-dose vitamin C (ascorbic acid) therapy to benefit patients with advanced cancer: A controlled trial," *New England Journal of Medicine* (1979) 301:687–90.

16. Michael J. Fay and Anthony J. Verlangieri, "Effects of calcium L-threonate on ascorbic acid uptake by human T-lymphocyte cells," *FASEB Journal* (Mar. 11, 1991) 5(4) A588, Abstract 1266.

17. Anthony J. Verlangieri, Anthony W. Bannon, and Michael J. Fay, "Anti-scorbutic activity of L-ascorbic acid and Ester-C in the non-ascorbate synthesizing ODS rat," *FASEB J.* (Mar. 11, 1991) 5(4) A588, Abstract 1265.

18. Anthony J. Verlangieri, Michael J. Fay, and Anthony W. Bannon, "Comparison of the anti-scorbutic activity of L-ascorbic acid and Ester-C in the non-ascorbate synthesizing Osteogenic Disorder Shionogi (ODS) rat," *Life Sciences* (June 10, 1991) 48(23) 2275–81.

CHAPTER 9

Vitamin E Against Cancer

Although I am discussing the antioxidant nutrients *separately,* please keep in mind that they work *synergistically.* That is, the protection they provide as a team is greater that the sum of the protection provided by each. A moderate balance of each antioxidant nutrient is far more effective than great quantities of a single antioxidant nutrient in the absence of one or more of the others.

The power of synergism can be well demonstrated by several studies involving vitamin E and other antioxidant nutrients. Selenium, the topic of the next chapter, is a trace mineral that is the key component of several antioxidant enzymes. A 1983 report on the synergistic effect of vitamin E and selenium on preventing breast cancer helped explain why the synergism occurs.[1] Drs. Paula Horvath and Clement Ip of what is now Buffalo's Roswell Park Cancer Institute found that "Vitamin E, although ineffective by itself, was able to potentiate the ability of selenium to inhibit the development of mammary tumors."

The researchers noted that although vitamin E was a potent antioxidant, it was not sufficient to inhibit tumor formation. Selenium alone was able to reduce tumor development, but not significantly. When adequate amounts of both vitamin E and selenium are present together, significant protection against tumor formation results. The researchers also noted that, "Our results indicate that vitamin E facilitates the anticarcinogenic action of selenium only when it is present during the promotion or proliferation phase."

The researchers concluded, "An adequate intake of antioxidants would obviously be advantageous, particularly in those consuming high levels of dietary fat, since diets rich in polyunsaturated fats are known to suppress certain immune functions."

Not all of the epidemiological studies show a positive effect of vitamin E, but most do. The above study illustrates why all don't. Looking at vitamin E by itself, or any antioxidant by itself, is a waste of time. What needs to be done is to look at the effect of all the antioxidants together. Researchers are now devising antioxidant nutrient indices to accomplish this.

In 1984, a team of British researchers led by Dr. N. J. Wald examined vitamin E and beta-carotene in the prevention of breast cancer. Blood had been collected from 5,004 women in Guernsey between 1968 and 1975, and stored frozen. By the end of 1982, 39 of these women developed breast cancer. Compared with a control group of other women of similar age, menopausal status, family history of cancer, and previous history of benign breast disease, the breast cancer victims had lower vitamin E levels in their blood.[2]

Dr. Wald concluded, "Vitamin E levels showed a statistically significant trend in risk—those with the lowest vitamin E levels having the highest risk of breast cancer." Overall, women who had vitamin E blood levels in the lowest 20 percent (quintile) of those tested had a five times higher risk of breast cancer than those whose vitamin E blood levels were in the highest 20 percent."

The average time from collection of the blood sample until breast cancer was detected was five years. This excludes the possibility that an undetected tumor affected the vitamin E blood level.

Beta-carotene levels tended to be lower in women who developed breast cancer. As Dr. Wald noted, "There was a suggestion of a trend for beta-carotene, but this was not statistically significant." The researchers had observed relationships between low blood vitamin E (independently) and beta-carotene (independently) and a high incidence of breast cancer. They did not look at the two nutrients as a team. What was the risk in those women who were exceedingly low in both vitamin E and beta-carotene compared to those who were well-nourished with both? From the study of Drs. Horvath and Ip, it is apparent that looking at vitamin E alone is missing the boat.

It wasn't until the following year that Dr. Jukka Salonen and his colleagues at the University of Kuopio (Finland) examined the roles of vitamin E and selenium together in preventing cancer. They had been studying over 12,000 Finns for several years in what is called the North Karelia Project. Four years after blood was drawn from these 12,155 persons, 51 had died of cancer. They were matched with others by age, sex and smoking habits, and their blood samples were compared.

In this study, many factors were examined, but most important, both vitamin E and selenium levels in the blood were examined in combination. The relative risk of cancer mortality for the third of people with blood selenium levels below 47 micrograms per liter of blood, compared to those with higher levels, was 5.8 to 1. But of more importance is the finding that, for persons with low selenium levels who also had vitamin E levels in the lowest values, risk of death from cancer compared to persons with both selenium and vitamin E levels in the upper two-thirds of values was 11.4 to 1.[3]

Looking at the figures another way, those in the top third of both vitamin E and selenium intakes had less than one-eleventh the cancer risk that those in the bottom third had. That is a reduction in cancer risk of 91 percent with intake of just those two antioxidant nutrients.

That proves my point that antioxidant nutrients can reduce your risk of cancer to one-tenth of the average risk! The figures would be even more dramatic if we compared the cancer incidences for people in the top tenth (decile) for both antioxidants to those in the bottom tenth for both. Your objective should be to eat enough fruits and vegetables or take appropriate supplements to put you in the top tenth for all of the antioxidant nutrients.

The importance of the relationship with selenium has been recognized by the National Research Center. Their 1989 booklet on "Diet and Health: Implications for reducing chronic disease risk" concluded "Low serum levels of vitamin E coupled with low selenium may increase the risks of at least some cancers such as breast and lung cancer."[4]

Now before leaving the role of vitamin E in cancer prevention, let's look at one study of vitamin E alone in reducing cancer risk. As I said earlier, this is missing the boat because it misses the synergistic effect, but since this is such a large study, it is important to look at.

In 1988, Finnish researchers reported on a ten-year follow-up of 21,172 men from six areas of Finland. Blood samples were drawn when the men entered the study. Subjects with possible signs of cancer at the time the blood samples were taken and those developing cancer within the first two years of follow-up were excluded from the study. Vitamin E levels were measured from the stored blood samples of 453 patients who developed cancer during the follow-up of six-to-ten years and 841 matched controls.

Study results showed that men with higher vitamin E levels had a lower cancer risk. The adjusted relative risks in the top 40 percent (two highest quintiles) of blood vitamin E levels had only 70 percent of the cancer risk of the remaining 60 percent, and only 60 percent of the risk of developing smoking-related cancers.[5] It's a shame these researchers didn't study both vitamin E and selenium at the same time.

Other Ways Vitamin E Prevents Cancer

Vitamin E does not act solely by destroying the free radicals that can initiate the cancer process. Vitamin E also interacts directly with some cancer-causing chemicals to inactivate them. Vitamin E, like vitamin C, prevents nitrates and nitrites from being converted into cancer-causing nitrosamines.

The amount of vitamin E required to optimize the immune system is greater than the 15 IU suggested as the RDA.[6] Less than optimal amounts of vitamin E result in poor T-cell and B-cell responses. Vitamin E supplements have been shown to enhance lymphocyte proliferation.[7]

Dr. Adrianne Bendich of Roche Center for Human Nutrition

in Nutley, New Jersey explains the importance of vitamin E to the immune system.

> "The generation of the immune response involves the interactions of white blood cells such as lymphocytes and mononuclear cells. These interactions include cell-to-cell communication, and the production of immunoreactive molecules (including interleukins, interferons, prostaglandins and leukotrienes). Essential activities also include lymphocyte proliferation and the synthesis and secretion of immunoglobulins (antibodies). . . . Vitamin E is important in maintaining the lymphocyte membrane fluidity necessary for the proliferative response."[8]

Research Summary

The Life Sciences Research Office of the Federation of American Societies for Experimental Biology examined the relationship of vitamin E and cancer for the Food and Drug Administration (FDA).[9] The 1992 report concluded,

> "Vitamin E has been suggested to play a role in several stages of carcinogenesis. These include a) inhibition or blockage of mutagen or carcinogen formation from precursors via direct chemical interaction, b) prevention of mutagens or carcinogens from reaching or reacting with DNA by scavenging mutagens or by enhancing detoxification processes, and c) prevention of cancer progression by the enhancement of normal immune responses.
> "In general, there are more studies suggesting a positive correlation between higher risk of cancers and lower intake or serum/plasma levels of vitamin E than those that do not fit this association."

My comment is that the few studies that missed the protective effect studied too few persons and should have looked at vitamin E and other antioxidants in combination.[10]

Prevention

The RDA for vitamin E for adults is 15 IU. It was reduced from 30 IU purely because dieticians could not readily design diets of the proper calorie levels that contained 30 IU. However, the RDA does not consider the role of vitamin E in the prevention of chronic diseases. What you should be interested in is the Optimal Daily Requirement.

You should consider getting at least 100 to 1,000 IU of vitamin E daily. The optimal range for most people is 400 to 800 IU. The important thing to remember about vitamin E is that you have to take it for a long time before you increase the cellular levels to the proper levels. It takes at least 60 to 90 days to achieve this anticancer effect.

Therapy

The importance of vitamin E to cancer patients is in enhancing the immune system so that the body can attack the cancer and prevent it from spreading.

Vitamin E should be administered as an adjunct therapy unless specifically contraindicated. One proven benefit of vitamin E is its ability to lessen the adverse effects of the chemotherapy drug Adriamycin, which include heart damage and baldness.[11] It is best to begin vitamin E supplementation before the drug is given if practical to do so. The more vitamin E that can enter cell membranes, the more the cells will be protected against the chemotherapy. Virtually all patients receiving Adriamycin lose their hair; however, nearly 70 percent of the patients receiving 1600 IU of vitamin E daily beginning several days before therapy did not suffer significant hair loss.[12]

REFERENCES

1. Paula M. Horvath and Clement Ip, "Synergistic effect of vitamin E and selenium in the chemoprevention of mammary carcinogenesis in rats," *Cancer Research* (Nov. 1983) 43:5335-41.

2. N. J. Wald et al., "Plasma retinol, beta-carotene and vitamin E levels in relation to the future risk of breast cancer," *British Journal of Cancer* (1984) 49:321–4.

3. Jukka T. Salonen et al., "Risk of cancer in relation to serum concentrations of selenium and vitamins A and E," *British Medical Journal* (Feb. 9, 1985) 290:417–20.

4. National Research Council, Committee on Diet, Nutrition and Cancer, "Diet and health: Implications for reducing chronic disease risk," (Washington, D.C.: National Academy Press, 1989).

5. P. Knekt et al., "Serum vitamin E and risk of cancer among Finnish men during a ten-year follow-up," *American Journal of Epidemiology* (1988) 127:28–41.

6. Adrianne Bendich, E. Gabriel, and Lawrence J. Machlin, "Dietary vitamin E requirement for optimum immune responses in the rat," *Journal of Nutrition* (1986) 116:675–81.

7. Adrianne Bendich, E. Gabriel, and Lawrence J. Machlin, "Effect of dietary level of vitamin E on the immune system," *Journal of Nutrition* (1983) 113:1920–6.

8. Adrianne Bendich, "Vitamin E and immunity," *Nutrition Report* (March 1987) 5(3)17, 21.

9. Ching K. Chow, "Evaluation of publicly available scientific evidence regarding certain nutrient-disease relationships: vitamin E and cancer," LSRO, FASEB, FDA Contract No. 223-88-2124 (Bethesda, MD: 1991).

10. Paul Knekt, "Role of vitamin E in the prophylaxis of cancer," *Annals of Medicine* (1991) 23:3–12.

11. J. Milei et al., "Amelioration of Adriamycin-induced cardiotoxicity in rabbits by prenylamine and vitamins A and E," *American Heart Journal* (1986) 111:95–102.

12. L. A. Wood, "Possible prevention of Adriamycin-induced alopecia by tocopherol," *New England Journal of Medicine* (April 18, 1985).

CHAPTER 10

Selenium Against Cancer

As was noted in the preceding chapter, selenium is a trace mineral that is an essential partner of vitamin E in the prevention of cancer. U.S. governmental agencies have recognized the role of selenium in preventing cancer in several official recommendations. There is also some preliminary evidence that selenium may play a vital role in the treatment of many malignant tumors.

As long ago as 1983 the National Research Council advised that "The results of a few epidemiological studies suggest a correlation between exposure to high levels of selenium and the reduction in the risk of certain cancers."[1] The following year, the National Institutes of Health recommended eating foods rich in antioxidants including vitamins A, C and E, and the trace mineral selenium.[2]

Selenium was a key element in my theories, publications and patents regarding cancer prevention in 1972. At that time, selenium was not known to be an essential nutrient for humans, nor was it known to be a component of any human biochemical compound. Selenium was of interest to me in my longevity studies because it had a synergistic effect with vitamin E in helping my laboratory animals live longer.

In the 1960s, all that we knew about the biochemistry of selenium was that it may have been a component of an unknown liver and kidney factor called "Factor-3" in chickens. I code-named my first longevity formula for my laboratory animals "Factor-3X" because of my emphasis on selenium. Surprisingly, few other scientists knew about the possible biochemical roles of selenium until 1973, when it was shown to be part of the important antioxidant enzyme, glutathione peroxidase.[3] Now selenium has been shown to be a part of at least two other human enzymes and several structural proteins.[4,5]

Selenium is now considered an essential human nutrient with an estimated desirable range of intake of 50 to 200 micrograms daily. Unfortunately, the amount of selenium in food depends on the selenium content of the soil, which varies from region to region and is disappearing from farmed soils (as it is not replaced, or on the content of selenium in feeds, which fortunately is being added to grow healthier animals. However, selenium usually decreases dramatically with the amount of processing applied to the food.

Hundreds of laboratory animal studies and dozens of epidemiological and case-controlled clinical studies have now shown that the better the selenium nutrition of a person, the less chance for cancer. The evidence includes prospective and retrospective clinical studies; epidemiological studies based on selenium content of food intake, blood, and soils; and laboratory animal studies that examined natural life spans, spontaneous cancers, carcinogen-induced (dietary, contact) cancers, virus-induced (both inoculated and not inoculated) cancers, transplanted cancer tissue, and inoculated cancer cells. Many cancer researchers are aware of the breadth and depth of the data.

The clinical confirmation that cancer probability correlates inversely with a person's blood selenium content (the higher the selenium, the less chance of cancer) was shown epidemiologically in the 1970s by Dr. Raymond Shamberger, and clinically in the 1980s by Dr. Walter Willett and his Harvard colleagues.[6,7]

There is no need to review hundreds of tests to make this point. I will mention six studies that make the point very well, and then describe an additional confirming study. I have reported on these studies before in the books *Selenium Update* and *The New Supernutrition,* but the information needs to be reiterated here.[8,9] This is what we learned from these six studies:

1. Considering blood selenium levels alone, those persons in the lowest fifth, when all subjects are ranked by blood selenium content, have twice the incidence of cancer as those in the highest fifth.[7]
2. Total cancer mortality is three times higher in persons having blood selenium levels below a certain value than the total cancer mortality in those above this value.[10]
3. Considering blood selenium levels alone, those persons in the lowest tenth of all blood selenium levels have six times the incidence of cancer as those in the highest tenth.[11]
4. Both selenium and vitamin E are needed together to prevent cancer.[12]
5. In regards to both selenium and vitamin E blood levels, those persons in the lowest third of all blood vitamin E levels who also had a low blood selenium level had more than 11 times the incidence of cancer as those in the upper two-thirds of blood vitamin E and selenium levels.[13]
6. Another study was published in which the researcher concluded that "selenium should be considered not only as a preventive, but also as a therapeutic agent in cancer treatment and may act additively or synergistically with drug and X-ray treatments."[14]

Selenium is involved in protecting the body against cancer in many ways. Selenium is a component of the antioxidant enzyme, glutathione peroxidase; it stimulates the immune system; it helps DNA repair itself; it reduces the action of carcinogens on DNA; it suppresses gene mutations; and it regulates certain enzyme interactions (as discussed in the previous chapter).

Study Details

You may find the details of the six studies of interest. If not, just skip ahead to the concluding section of this chapter. Here are brief summaries of the six studies plus one confirming study for good measure.

THE WILLETT STUDY

This study is of major importance, not only for its research, but for its influence. The Willett study was conducted by a well-respected group of researchers, and the work was done at major centers of learning: Harvard, Johns Hopkins, Duke, the University of Texas, and other respected universities. The results were published in a major medical journal, rather than an obscure scientific periodical. Many physicians read of the importance of blood selenium levels and their relationship to cancer risk for the first time, thanks to this study.

In the Willett study, blood samples had been collected in 1973 from 4,480 men from 14 regions of the United States. At the time of collection of the blood samples, none of the men had detectable signs of cancer. The blood samples were preserved and stored for later analyses.

During the next five years, 111 cases of cancer were detected in this group. The researchers then retrieved the stored blood samples from these men, and from 210 other men who were selected because they matched the newly developed cancer patients in age, race, sex, and smoking history. The levels of several nutrients and other factors were compared between the men who developed cancer and those men who remained free of cancer.

One difference stood out as being highly significant. The risk of cancer for subjects in the lowest fifth was *twice* that of subjects in the highest fifth.[7]

Dr. Willett's group reviewed the evidence of the association of low blood selenium levels and cancer at a symposium in 1990, whereby the results were published the following year.[15]

THE CHINESE STUDY

This study, examining the relationship between blood levels of selenium in 1,458 healthy adults in 24 regions of China, was led by Dr. Shu-Yu Yu of the Cancer Institute of the Chinese Academy of Medical Sciences in Beijing. The researchers found that there was a statistically significant inverse correlation between age-adjusted cancer death rates and the selenium levels of the blood of local residents. In the areas with high selenium levels, there was significantly lower cancer mortality in both males and females. Total cancer mortality was three times higher in areas where the mean blood selenium level was greater than 11 micrograms per deciliter of blood then where it was 8 micrograms per deciliter.[10]

Dr. Shu-Yu Yu confirmed these results in studies that were reported three years lager.[16,17]

THE CLARK STUDY

Dr. Larry Clark and colleagues at Cornell University determined the blood selenium levels in 240 skin cancer patients and compared the results to those from 103 apparently healthy persons living in low-selenium areas. The mean blood selenium level for the skin cancer patients was significantly lower than that of the apparently healthy individuals. After adjusting for age, sun damage to the skin, blood beta-carotene and vitamin A levels, and other factors, the incidence of skin cancer in those persons in the lowest tenth of blood selenium levels was 5.8 times as great as those in the top tenth.[11]

It should be noted that selenium, in the form of the common food supplement L-selenomethionine, can protect skin against sun-induced damage.[18] Interestingly, the selenium compound protects whether taken orally or applied to the skin.

THE HORVATH STUDY

The preceding studies have dealt with real people, but let's look at an important laboratory animal study for a moment. Most scientific experiments examine one variable at a time to study the effect of just that one variable. This reduces confusion from confounding factors. Yet, the body is not a simple laboratory! It is a biologically complex mechanism that functions independently of science's effort to study it.

I have stressed the biological synergism of all the antioxidant nutrients, but I do so especially of vitamin E and selenium. In the preceding chapter, I discussed the study published by Drs. Paula

Horvath and Clement Ip that showed that both vitamin E and selenium must be present *together* to prevent the proliferative phase of cancer. Their evidence indicates that it is not the amount of the selenium-containing enzyme (glutathione peroxidase) that is critical, but the amount of another enzyme, microsomal peroxidase, which is stimulated only when both vitamin E and selenium are present together.[12]

The message here is that scientists should not be studying the correlation between blood selenium levels alone and cancer, but they should be studying the correlation between blood levels of selenium and vitamin E together. Studying selenium alone, we do, in fact, find that there is a substantial reduction in cancer risk with the higher blood selenium levels. We find the same relationship with vitamin E and some types of cancer, as we noted in the preceding chapter. However, when a person's blood is rich in both selenium and vitamin E, the protection given that person is far more than that of adding the selenium protection and the vitamin E protection together.

If a person has a normal blood level of vitamin E, but is *very* deficient in selenium, that person will not have a good defense against cancer. Conversely, if a person is a *little* low in vitamin E, but well-fortified with selenium, then that person may be more resistant to cancer.

Since the vitamin E level of the blood can affect the usefulness of selenium, researchers should be looking at the combined levels—not just simply one or the other. Once researchers catch on to this concept, we will see more dramatic results. This becomes apparent in the next study.

The Finnish Study

Dr. Jukka Salonen and his colleagues at the University of Kuopio in Finland have been studying over 12,000 Finns for several years. The study is known as the North Karlia Project. Four years after blood samples were drawn from these 12,155 persons, 51 had died of cancer. They were matched for age, sex and smoking habits with others, and the results of their blood samples were compared.

In this study, many factors were examined, but most important, both vitamin E and selenium levels of the blood were examined in combination. The relative risk of cancer mortality for the third of people with blood selenium levels below 47 micrograms per liter of blood compared to those with higher levels was 5.8 to 1. But of greater importance is the finding that for people with low selenium levels who also had vitamin E levels in the lowest range, the *risk of death from cancer compared to persons having blood levels of both selenium and vitamin E in the upper two-thirds of values was 11.4 to 1.*

THE MILNER REVIEW

Dr. John A. Milner of the University of Illinois has been studying selenium and cancer protection for about two decades. Most of Dr. Milner's studies involve transplanting or inoculating cancer cells into mice receiving different levels of selenium in their food or drinking water. He has found that selenium inhibits the development of such cancers.

Dr. Milner's conclusion is that selenium should be considered not only as a preventive, but also as a therapeutic agent in cancer treatment.[15] There is also some evidence that selenium may act additively or synergistically with drug and/or radiation treatments.

In addition to Dr. Milner's review, Drs. Gerald Combs and Larry Clark of Cornell presented an excellent review of selenium's protective roles against cancer in the November 1985 issue of *Nutrition Reviews*. They provided 97 references for the serious scholar to pursue. At this writing there are now over 400 related articles on the role of selenium in cancer prevention.

Cancer Therapy

In the early 1970s, when it was clear that optimal intake of selenium was protective against cancer in laboratory animals, Dr. Gerhard Schrauzer of the University of California at San Diego and I called for clinical trials to test for this capability in humans. Dr.

Schrauzer had completed a series of experiments that showed that optimal selenium intake could reduce the natural occurrence of breast cancer in mice by nearly 90 percent, to only 12 percent of the usual cancer rate.[19] He told the National Cancer Institute in 1978 that the key to cancer prevention lies in assuring adequate selenium intake.

Dr. Schrauzer stated in a 1978 article in *Family Circle* magazine that if every woman in America started taking selenium (supplements) today, or had a high-selenium diet, within a few years the breast cancer rate would decline drastically. He also remarked that if a breast cancer patient has low selenium levels in her blood, her tendency to develop metastases (other tumors spread from the first) is increased, her possibility for survival is diminished, and her prognosis in general is poorer than if she had normal blood selenium levels.

In 1983, I reported in the first update of this book the encouraging results of Dr. Richard Donaldson of the St. Louis Veterans Administration Hospital. Dr. Donaldson passed away before he could complete his studies or publish his preliminary results, but this information should be reported again.

Dr. Donaldson did orally present his data to the National Cancer Institute, involving the first 140 patients enrolled in his study. According to Dr. Donaldson's letters, all the patients who entered the study were certified as being terminally ill by two physicians after receiving the appropriate conventional therapy for their particular cancer. Some of the patients who entered the program with only weeks to live were alive and well after four years, and with no signs or symptoms of cancer. Not all patients were cured, but all had reduction in tumor size and pain. It is unfortunate that they did not receive the selenium until they were pronounced incurable. This research may well change cancer therapy in the future.

It is important to realize that the dramatic improvements did not occur until sufficient selenium was ingested to bring the patient's blood selenium level up to normal. Sometimes this could be achieved in a few weeks with 200 to 600 micrograms of selenium per day, while other individuals required as much as 2,000 micrograms of selenium per day to normalize the blood selenium levels.

The critical factor is to have a physician monitor blood selenium levels. Since not every laboratory can analyze blood for selenium content, the physician may have to send the blood samples to regional laboratories. Physicians wishing more information as to the preferred blood selenium level for cancer patients may wish to write directly to Dr. Schrauzer.

In Dr. Donaldson's clinical trials, no signs of selenium toxicity were observed in any patient—even in the autopsies of the 37 patients who were helped, but not cured by the therapy. It should be pointed out that other antioxidant nutrients, including vitamins A, C and E, were also used in Dr. Donaldson's program.

Selenium Supplementation

The important aspect of selenium nutrition is that it is the amount of selenium in the blood and tissues that counts. There appears to be a threshold level that must be maintained in the blood in order for the body to produce adequate amounts of the antioxidant enzymes, the selenium-containing peroxidases.

Since selenium-containing foods can vary in selenium content by over a thousandfold, depending on where the plants were grown or what the animals were fed, it is apparent that one should not trust book values for estimating the selenium content of the diet. In my opinion, the only practical way to ensure that you get adequate amounts of selenium is to take selenium supplements. Supplements are measured amounts of nutrients.

The "official" recommended range for selenium is 50 to 200 micrograms per day. I feel that this is too low, and that 400 to 500 micrograms daily would more closely approximate the intake of the low-cancer populations of Japan, who consume about 600 micrograms daily. This also approximates the extrapolation of Dr. Schrauzer, which indicates that this level would lower the cancer incidence to just above the no-incidence level.

Assuming that you do get some selenium in your diet, you may wish to consider taking 200 (or even as much as 400) micrograms daily as a supplement. Cancer patients may wish to take 600 micrograms daily as a supplement.

However, selenium, like almost all substances, is toxic in excess. It is important to remember that the toxic level for selenium begins just above the safe range of 1,000 micrograms per day. This may be lower for some persons and for some forms of selenium. Unless your blood level of selenium is monitored by a physician, do not exceed the above-mentioned levels.

REFERENCES

1. *Diet, Nutrition, and Cancer: Directions for research,* Committee on Diet, Nutrition, and Cancer, (Washington, D.C.: National Academy Press, 1983).
2. *Diet, Nutrition & Cancer Prevention,* National Institutes of Health, Public Health Service, U.S. Department of Health & Human Services, NIH Publ. No. 85-2711 (Nov. 1984).
3. J. T. Rotruck, A. L. Pope et al., "Selenium: Biochemical role as a component of glutathione peroxidase," *Science* (1973) 179(73):588–90.
4. F. Ursini, M. Maiorino and C. Gregolin, "The selenoenzyme phospholipid hydroperoxide glutathione peroxidase," *Biochem. Biophys. Acta* (1985) 839(1):62–70.
5. M. J. Berry, L. Bann and P. R. Larsen, "Type I iodothyronine deiodinase is a selenocysteine-containing enzyme," *Nature* (1991) 349(6308):438–40.
6. Raymond J. Shamberger and C. E. Willis, "Selenium distribution and human cancer mortality," CRC Crit. Rev. Clin. Lab. Sci. (1971) 2(2):211–21.
7. W. C. Willett et al., "Prediagnostic serum selenium and risk of cancer," *Lancet* (July 16, 1983) II:130–4.
8. Richard A. Passwater, *Selenium Update,* (New Canaan, Conn: Keats Publishing, Inc., 1987).
9. Richard A. Passwater, *The New Supernutrition,* (New York: Pocket Books, 1991).
10. Shu-Yu Yu et al., "Regional variation of cancer mortality incidence and its relation to selenium levels in China," *Biological Trace Element Research* (Jan.–Feb. 1985) 7:21–9.

11. Lawrence C. Clark et al., "Plasma selenium and skin neoplasms: A case-controlled study," *Nutrition & Cancer* (Jan.–March 1984) 6:13–21.
12. Paula M. Horvath and Clement Ip, "Synergistic effect of vitamin E and selenium in the chemoprevention of mammary carcinogenesis in rats," *Cancer Research* (Nov. 1983) 43:5335–41.
13. Jukka T. Salonen, "Risk of cancer in relation to serum concentrations of selenium and vitamins A and E," *British Medical Journal* (Feb. 9, 1985) 290:417–20.
14. John A. Milner, "Selenium and the transplantable tumor," *Journal of Agricultural and Food Chemistry* (May–June 1984) 32:436–42.
15. Walter C. Willett et al., "The epidemiology of selenium and human cancer," In: Antero Aitio, editor, *Proceedings of the Joint Nordic Trace Element Society*/Union of Pure and Applied Chemistry International Symposium 1990. (1991) 141–55.
16. Shu-Yu Yu, Y. J. Chu, and W. G. Li, "Selenium chemoprevention of liver cancer in animals and possible human applications," *Biolog. Trace Element Res.* (1988) 15:231–41.
17. Shu-Yu Yu et al., "Biochemical and cellular aspects of the anticancer activity of selenium," *Biolog. Trace Element Res.* (1988) 15:243–55.
18. Karen E. Burke, "Skin cancer protection with L-selenomethionine," *Nutrition Report* (Oct. 1992) 10(10):73,80.
19. Gerhard Schrauzer and D. Ishmael, *Annals of Clinical and Laboratory Science* (1974) 4:441–7.

CHAPTER 11

Sulfur-Containing Antioxidants

The antioxidant nutrients discussed in the previous chapters are the most critical because they are the ones in shortest supply in the diet. However, the bulk of antioxidant nutrients are needed to help keep these scarcer nutrients in their active state. The body uses sulfur compounds called *thiols* to achieve this recharging and recycling of the trace antioxidants. These sulfur compounds also are potent antioxidants themselves.

My original research used the sulfur-containing amino acids methionine and cysteine, and the tripeptide glutathione extensively. Now we are aware of additional powerful sulfur-containing nutrients to help us.

Sulfur nutrients tend to have distinctive odors. Foods such as garlic, onions, cabbage, and eggs are rich in sulfur nutrients. You may also wish to include sulfur-containing nutrients in your supplementation program.

Lipoic Acid

Lipoic acid (also called thiotic acid) is a powerful antioxidant that may become an important nutrient by the late 1990s. It is not now considered essential for humans, as we can make some in our bodies—but can we make enough for optimum health?

Several researchers are studying the advantages of supplementation with lipoic acid, and this nutrient should become of increasing interest in the next few years.

Glutathione

Glutathione is the body's major antioxidant and is normally produced in ample quantities provided one eats ample sulfur-containing foods, especially those rich in cysteine or cystine. Glutathione is well-absorbed and readily enters cells to work as an antioxidant—except in AIDS patients. AIDs patients lose immune function because their cells can't make enough glutathione internally, and glutathione made outside of the deficient cells or absorbed from food is not transported across cells infected with HIV (the AIDS virus).

However, another sulfur-containing nutrient, NAC (N-acetylcysteine) can penetrate HIV-infected cells and produce significant amounts of glutathione so as to restore significant immune function.

N-acetylcysteine (NAC)

N-acetylcysteine (NAC) is found in small quantities in several foods, but the most reliable source is NAC supplements. NAC is of interest to researchers for its antioxidant effects in preventing cancer and reducing harmful lipoprotein (alpha) levels which are a factor in heart disease. It is also of interest in AIDS research.

Cysteine, Cystine and Methionine

These sulfur-containing amino acids are present in most sulfur-rich foods, and are also available as food supplements.

Garlic

Garlic is a rich source of sulfur compounds, including the powerful antioxidants ajone and dithiins, and other thiols. The world's garlic-eating peoples have lower cancer incidences than those who do not make the herb a regular part of their diet.

Sulfur-containing nutrients used to be in favor with the old-time nutritionists, but it will take modern nutritionists some time yet to catch up with the science of these protective nutrients. I feel that you will be reading quite a lot about sulfur-containing nutrients in the years to come as they are rediscovered.

CHAPTER 12

Trace Minerals, Antioxidant Enzymes and Pro-Oxidants

Earlier chapters have covered the major antioxidant nutrients, vitamin A and beta-carotene, vitamin C, vitamin E, the trace mineral selenium and sulfur-containing nutrients. These are the nutrients that you can take to reduce free-radical damage. However, your body makes additional complex antioxidant enzymes to protect itself, and nutrients are needed for the body to manufacture these enzymes.

I have already described how selenium itself is not an antioxidant, but that your body makes antioxidant enzymes, the peroxidases, using selenium as a key component. The peroxidases destroy free radicals called peroxides. When other free radicals attack the fats (lipids) in our cell membranes, new and very harmful free radicals are formed called lipid peroxides. Therefore, dietary selenium is essential for your antioxidant defense.

Other trace minerals are also important for the antioxidant enzymes that the body forms from them. The trace minerals zinc, copper and manganese are part of the antioxidant enzyme called superoxide dismutase (SOD). SOD converts the oxygen-free radical, superoxide, into the less harmful peroxide, hydrogen peroxide.

Therefore, if we are deficient in zinc, copper or manganese, we will not produce adequate SOD and free radical damage from superoxide radicals can occur.

Iron is essential for many reasons, but of special interest to us in cancer prevention is that iron is part of the antioxidant enzyme catalase. Catalase converts hydrogen peroxide into water. Thus, we need SOD and catalase for optimal protection against superoxide radicals. If we are iron deficient, we aren't as well protected as we could be.

Pro-oxidants

It is not that simple, however! Iron and copper are also pro-oxidants. That is, iron and copper, when in the blood and tissues as free ions and not protected by proteins or serving as parts of compounds, react with body components to form free radicals. They are needed to protect against free radicals, but in excess, they can also cause free radicals.

During the next few years, my research will concentrate on finding the optimal amounts of each for optimal health, including prevention of cancer and heart disease. Until more research is available, the best recommendation appears to be to strive for the RDA for each trace mineral and not under-supply or over-supply your diet with any trace mineral. There is also another complication.

Competition and Balance

Trace mineral balance is essential. Many trace minerals compete with one another for absorption and transport. If you take too much of one trace mineral you may lessen the absorption of another. This is especially true for zinc and copper. Calcium also blocks the absorption of zinc, copper and selenium, yet we need adequate amounts of calcium as I will discuss in Chapter 14.

This may also explain why the epidemiological studies are showing that copper deficiency is associated with higher cancer risk, and an *excess* of copper is also associated with a higher cancer risk. The same is true so far for zinc; zinc deficiency is associated with higher cancer risk and zinc excess is also associated with higher cancer risk. Or the variance may be merely due to study variations in the methods.

Immune Response

These trace minerals are important for the antioxidant enzymes that they form, but they are also important in your cancer defense because they affect the immune response. Selenium, zinc and copper all are key nutrients for a healthy immune response. A zinc deficiency impairs the immune response, but it appears that an excess of zinc also impairs the immune response. Would that be because too much zinc interferes with the absorption of copper, which is also needed for a healthy immune system?

Recommended Amounts

In review, the trace minerals zinc, copper, manganese and iron are critical for cancer prevention. However, too much out of balance may be as detrimental as too little. Follow the RDAs.

Here are the 1989 RDAs:

zinc (men)	15 mg (elemental)
(women)	12 mg (elemental)
copper	1.5–3 mg (elemental)
manganese	2–5 mg (elemental)
iron (men)	10 mg (elemental)
(women)	15 mg (elemental)

CHAPTER 13

Vitamin B Complex Against Cancer

So far, we have discussed the major antioxidant nutrients and how they prevent cancer by destroying cancer-causing free radicals. Although some of the B-complex vitamins are minor antioxidants, their functions are to form the coenzymes that in turn form many of the thousands of enzymes that make your body chemistry work.

However, there is more to cancer protection than destroying the free-radical aggressors. You must also maintain the health of your DNA and immune system. Your DNA is the protein factory that repairs and reproduces your vital components. DNA molecules are linked together to form the genetic material, the chromosomes. If your DNA is damaged, it may produce mutations of your cells instead of exact copies. If you allow poor nutrition to weaken your DNA, then the DNA becomes faulty even if there is no free-radical aggressor at all. Free radicals can harm healthy DNA, but poor nutrition can bring about the same result and lead to cancer.

Cancer protection requires that first of all, you are well-nourished. Secondly, you must protect yourself from the inevitable free radicals that always are in your body no matter how "careful" you try to be, and thirdly, you should avoid overexposure to free-radical sources.

The B-complex vitamin, folic acid (also called folate, folacin or pteroylglutamic acid), is required for healthy DNA. In fact, it often is the weak link—and even missing link—in DNA health. As *Nutrition Reviews* puts it, "Folic acid deficiency is associated with a variety of chromosomal abnormalities. Chromosome breaks, gaps, despiralization and increased sister chromatid exchanges have been reported in the setting of folate deficiency."[1]

In other words, a variety of types of DNA damage can occur when there is a folic acid deficiency that will not occur when there is adequate folic acid nutriture. A common example that has been often cited is that caffeine produces chromosomal damage when there is a folic acid deficiency, but doesn't when there is adequate folic acid nutriture.[1]

Thus, it is not surprising to learn that folic acid deficiency at conception leads to a greater risk of birth defects.[2] The bad news is, most Americans do not get adequate amounts of folic acid. In fact, many nutritionists feel that folic acid deficiency is our number-one vitamin deficiency.[1,3]

Dr. Charles E. Butterworth, Jr. and his colleagues at the University of Alabama Medical School have linked folic acid deficiency to both cervical cancer and lung cancer. They reported in the *Journal of the American Medical Association* that women with a deficiency of folic acid were five times more likely than others to develop the precancerous cell growth known as cervical dysplasia when exposed to the human papilloma virus.[4] This will be discussed later in Chapter 23 on Cervical Cancer. It is interesting to note that when women taking oral contraceptives have Pap smear tests showing the presence of precancerous dysplastic cells, merely improving the folic acid nutriture quickly normalizes the results of the Pap smear test.[5]

Dr. Butterworth's group also reported that vitamin B12 and folic acid together appear to reverse or decrease precancerous changes in the lungs of cigarette smokers. Smokers treated for four months with high doses of these two B-complex vitamins showed significant improvement in the number of precancerous cells in sputum from their lungs. The study involved 88 men who smoked at least a pack a day for 20 years or more, and was confirmed by a later study.[6,7]

Dr. Butterworth said that the treatment was "a poor substitute for stopping smoking," but added that "this may enable doctors to prevent premalignant growths from developing into lung cancer. We think this is very encouraging evidence, first to support the concept of localized vitamin deficiency, and second, it may help explain some of the underlying mechanisms by which cells are altered genetically."

Choline and DMG

A deficiency of choline may also initiate cancer. Choline is not considered an official vitamin for humans because we can make some choline from the amino acid methionine. However, many researchers feel that we may not always be able to make as much choline as we should for optimum health, and they group choline "unofficially" in with the B-complex family of vitamins.

What we are really concerned with is the availability of a portion of the molecule normally supplied by the essential amino acid called a "methyl group." The body does not synthesize methyl groups and depends on the diet for these groups of atoms. These pre-arranged atoms are needed to make many compounds including choline.

We depend primarily on our total intake of methionine, choline, dimethylglycine (DMG) and betaine (trimethylglycine) for the labile (easily used) methyl groups needed for transmethylation (donated methyl groups for our body's needs).

Dr. Lionel Poirier of the National Center for Toxicological Research Division of the Food and Drug Administration reported at an American Institute for Cancer Research Conference that "a scarcity of methyl groups can change the structure of the DNA molecule, leading to breaks and rearrangements that can profoundly affect the genetic machinery of the cell. One of the results may be cancer."[8]

A deficiency of choline plus the other methyl group donors can induce cancer even in the absence of carcinogens and/or free radicals. Researchers at the University of Toronto fed rats a diet low in choline and methionine and found precancerous changes in their livers within ten weeks. Choline supplementation prevented these precancerous changes.[9]

Dimethylglycine (DMG) has been found to be a potent stimulator of both branches of the immune system.[10,11]

REFERENCES

1. "Folate deficiency, parenteral caffeine, and cytogenic damage in mice," *Nutrition Reviews* (Sept. 1991) 49(9):285–7.
2. K. M. Laurence et al., "Double-blind randomized controlled trial of folate treatment before conception to prevent recurrence of neural-tube defects," *British Medical Journal* (1981) 282:1509–11.
3. I. Eto and A. Sancar, "Role of vitamin B-12 and folate deficiencies in carcinogenesis," In: *Essential nutrients in carcinogenesis*. L. A. Poirer, M. W. Pariza, and P. M. Newberne, eds. (NY: Plenum Press, 1986), 313–30.
4. C. E. Butterworth, Jr.; K. D. Hatch et al., "Folate deficiency and cervical dysplasia," *JAMA* (1992) 267(4):528–33.
5. C. E. Butterworth et al., "Improvement of cervical dysplasia associated with folic acid therapy in users of oral contraceptives," *American Journal of Clinical Nutrition* (1982) 35:73–82.
6. "B vitamins help reduce squamous metaplasia in smokers," *The Record* (1986) 12/4.
7. D. C. Heimburger et al., "Improvement in bronchial squamous metaplasia in smokers treated with folate and vitamin B-12," *Journal of the American Medical Association* (1988) 259:1525–30.
8. Lionel Poirier, "Research Update: Probing the effects of methyl deficiency," *American Institute of Cancer Research Newsletter* (Summer 1991) #32.
9. A. Ghoshal, T. Rushmore, and E. Farber, "Initiation of carcinogenesis by a dietary deficiency of choline in the absence of added carcinogens," *Cancer Letters* (1987) 36:289–96.
10. E. A. Reap and J. W. Lawson, "Stimulation of the immune response by dimethylglycine, a nontoxic metabolite," *J. Lab. Clin. Med.* (1990) 115(4):481–6.
11. C. D. Graber, J. M. Goust, et al., "Immunomodulating properties of dimethylglycine in humans," *J. Infect. Disease* (1981) 143(1):101–5.

CHAPTER 14

Vitamin D and Calcium Protect Against Some Cancers

Few suspected a link—direct or indirect—between vitamin D and cancer prevention, but lo and behold there is. In 1988, Drs. Cedric F. Garland and Frank C. Garland of the University of California School of Medicine at San Diego published a book entitled *The Calcium Connection*. This book deals with their studies of the relationship between vitamin D and calcium and preventing breast and colon cancers.

In 1979, they were attending a lecture at Johns Hopkins University that included maps showing the incidence of each of the major cancers for each of the 3,056 counties in the U.S. These maps were prepared by Dr. T. J. Mason and his colleagues at the National Cancer Institute from data supplied by the National Center for Health Statistics. I published some of these maps in the first edition of *Cancer and Its Nutritional Therapies,* and they are repeated here for your convenience.

Note, by looking at the fifth and last map, "Melanoma," that it is obvious that people living in warmer climates have more exposure to the sun and thus more overexposure to ultraviolet energy; thus, people living in warmer climates have more skin

cancer. Now look at the third figure, "Breast cancer, white females." Do you see a pattern?

Dr. Cedrick Garland did. He noticed that it looked as if some-
one had drawn a heavy line along the 40th parallel—through the
middle of California, and the tops of Arizona, New Mexico, Texas,
Tennessee and the Carolinas. The vast majority of the high breast
cancer areas are North of this line while most of the low breast
cancer areas are South of it. The same is true of the map for colon
(large intestine) cancer.

For both cancers, there is a correlation showing a decreasing
gradient of mortality rates from North to South. "At first we
thought that the link was due to differences in the diet between
the North and South, but when we look at data from the Department of Agriculture, we found that (no dietary pattern) fitted the
map we had produced for cancer."[1]

The next obvious explanation would be exposure to sunlight.
The warmer the climate, the more skin exposure to sunlight. The
more sunlight reaching the skin, the more vitamin D that the body
forms in the skin from cholesterol-derived compounds. So the
scientists decided to look at the possible role of vitamin D.

Where there were some apparent exceptions to the map pattern—in large cities in the South, these can also be explained by
the sunlight theory. People living in large cities live in polluted air
that blocks sunlight and live in the shadows of tall buildings. Also,
city folk tend not to wear short-sleeve shirts and shorts as often as
country folk, and they tend not to be outside in the sunniest hours.
The Drs. Garland published their hypothesis in 1980.[2]

In 1984, the Drs. Garland convinced some of the researchers mentioned in Chapter 7, who looked into the effects of vitamin A and
beta-carotene on lung cancer, to use their data bank and blood samples
to look into calcium and/or vitamin D and colon cancer. The researchers, originally led by Drs. Richard Shekelle and Jeremiah
Stamler, conducted the Western Electric Study wherein 1,954 men
living near Chicago volunteered to be studied over 20 years.

The researchers found that the risk of colon cancer was inversely
correlated with dietary vitamin D and calcium. When the combined intakes of vitamin D and calcium were ranked, and then

grouped as "fourths" or "quartiles" from lowest to highest intakes, the observed risks were 38.9, 24.5, 22.5 and 14.3 per 1,000 population. This association remained significant after adjustment for age, cigarette smoking, body mass index, alcohol consumption, and percentage of calories obtained from fat.[3]

The study found that a dietary intake of vitamin D greater than 3.75 micrograms of vitamin D per day was associated with a 50 percent reduction in the incidence of colorectal cancer, and that a dietary intake of 1200 milligrams or more per day of calcium was associated with a 75 percent reduction.

The Drs. Garland and their colleagues continued to look into this possible relationship. Later they reported that "people who get at least 400 IUs of vitamin D daily are half as likely to get colon cancer as those who get less."[4] Dr. Garland also suggested that "breast cancer rates could be significantly cut by a diet rich in vitamin D."[4]

In 1989, Dr. Garland explained, "It appears that cancer is prevented because you need vitamin D to absorb calcium, and calcium inhibits cells from proliferating and becoming cancerous. . . . We're confident that increasing dietary vitamin D will reduce the overall incidence of breast and colon cancer."[1]

In 1990, Dr. Garland added, "Recent European studies of the metabolic roles of vitamin D indicate that when an adequate amount of vitamin D is present, the cells bind together tightly. Cells that are tightly bound together grow in a very regulated way. Individual cells are then less able to run out of control. When vitamin D is lacking, the binding loosens, leaving the cancer-prone cells to grow uncontrolled. The result is often cancer."[1]

An eight-year study of 25,802 Maryland residents found that people with blood levels of vitamin D that correlate to 400 IU or more daily of vitamin D had half the risk of colon cancer of those with lower amounts of vitamin D in their blood.[4] The cancer rate was three times higher for those who had less than the amount of vitamin D in the blood equivalent to an intake of 270 IU daily.

The researchers examined the breast cancer and colon cancer rates in 29 U.S. cities and 20 Canadian cities and found that the greater the amount of sunlight-blocking air pollution, the higher the breast cancer and colon cancer rates.[4]

Dr. Garland's research group also reported a threefold increase in the incidence of breast cancer in the republics of what was formerly called the Soviet Union, where there are low sunshine levels.[1]

We will again discuss the roles of vitamin D and calcium in Chapters 19 and 20 on Breast Cancer and Colon Cancer respectively. Researchers can find a good review of vitamin D and mechanisms for cancer prevention in reference 7.

Calcium

We don't really know if it is the vitamin D, the calcium, or both vitamin D and calcium working together that is protective. Since the major protective factor could be calcium, let's look at some of the supporting evidence.

Dr. Cedrick Garland presented his evidence to Drs. Martin Lipkin and Harold Newmark at the Memorial Sloan-Kettering Cancer Center in New York City. Drs. Lipkin and Newmark were studying persons at high risk for colon cancer due to their family histories of high incidences of colon cancer.

Drs. Lipkin and Newmark found that these high-risk persons, before taking calcium supplements, had an unusually high rate of cell proliferation (cell division) in their colons. After taking 1250 milligrams of calcium carbonate daily for two to three months, the rate of cell division returned to normal.[5]

Drs. Lipkin and Newmark now conclude that "calcium contributes to the progression of epithelial cells through all phases of the proliferative cycle and into stages of cell differentiation; intercellular concentrations of calcium that are required for cell renewal, however, are lower than those required for epithelial-cell differentiation. These effects of calcium are modulated by interactions with vitamin D, phosphate, and fats, all of which are dependent on dietary intake."[6]

Thus, low calcium intakes cause epithelial cells to proliferate but not differentiate (mature) to become normal cells. Fat increases this proliferation, but it can be overcome with adequate calcium intake. "Increased dietary calcium inhibits hyperproliferation of colon epithelial cells induced by increased levels of fats or bile acids in the colon. When carcinogens induce hyperproliferation of colon epithelial cells, the hyperproliferation is decreased by adding dietary calcium."[7]

We will look into the practicalities of this relationship again in the chapters on breast cancer and lung cancer.

How Much?

The 1989 adult RDA for vitamin D is 200 IU per day. Dr. Garland suggests that 400 IU is both safe and protective. Problems from too much vitamin D don't appear until 1,000 IU or more daily.

The adult 1989 RDA for calcium is 800 milligrams per day. You may wish to take a supplement containing 800 milligrams of calcium (elemental) in addition to the calcium in your normal diet.

REFERENCES

1. "Natural vitamin D helps reduce risk of cancer," *Nutrition Week* (March 1, 1990) 20(9):8.
2. Cedrick F. Garland and Frank C. Garland, "Do sunlight and vitamin D reduce the likelihood of colon cancer?" *International Journal of Epidemiology* (1980) 9(3):227–31.
3. Cedrick F. Garland et al., "Dietary vitamin D and calcium and the risk of colorectal cancer: a 19-year prospective study in men," *Lancet* (Feb. 5, 1985) I(8424):307–9.
4. Marilyn Elias, "Vitamin D may help beat cancer," *USA Today* (Jan. 26, 1989).
5. S. Manolagus, "Vitamin D and its relevance to cancer," *Anticancer Research* (1987) 7:625–38.
6. Martin Lipkin and Harold Newmark, "Effect of added dietary calcium on colonic epithelial-cell proliferation in subjects at high risk for familial colonic cancer," *New England Journal of Medicine* (Nov. 28, 1985) 313(22):1381–4.
7. Harold L. Newmark and Martin Lipkin, "Calcium, vitamin D and colon cancer," *Cancer Research* (April 1992) 52 (7 Suppl):2067s–2070s.

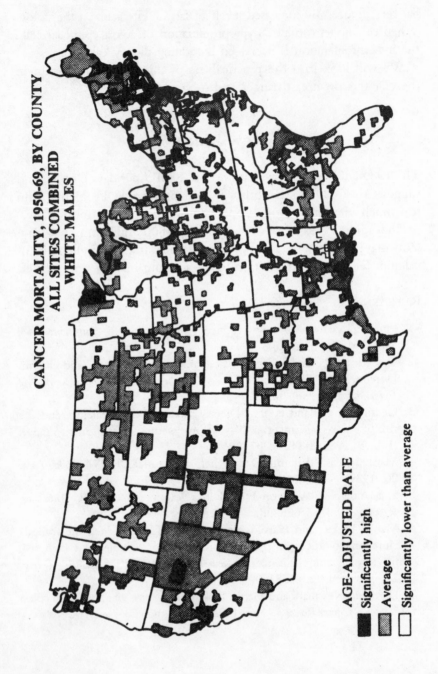

CANCER MORTALITY, 1950-69, BY COUNTY
ALL SITES COMBINED
WHITE MALES

AGE-ADJUSTED RATE

■ Significantly high

▨ Average

□ Significantly lower than average

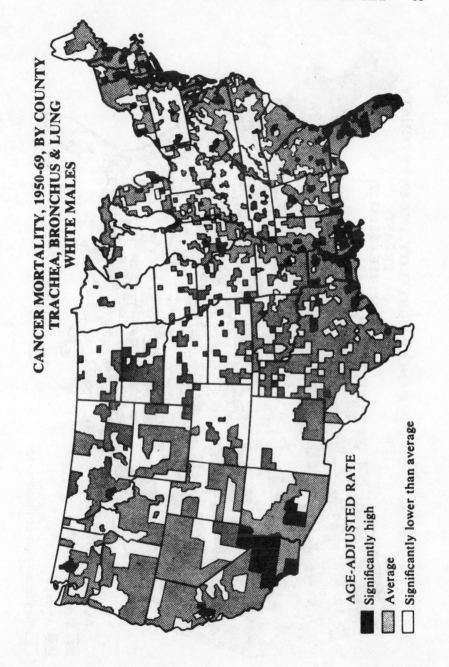

CANCER MORTALITY, 1950-69, BY COUNTY
TRACHEA, BRONCHUS & LUNG
WHITE MALES

AGE-ADJUSTED RATE

■ Significantly high

▨ Average

□ Significantly lower than average

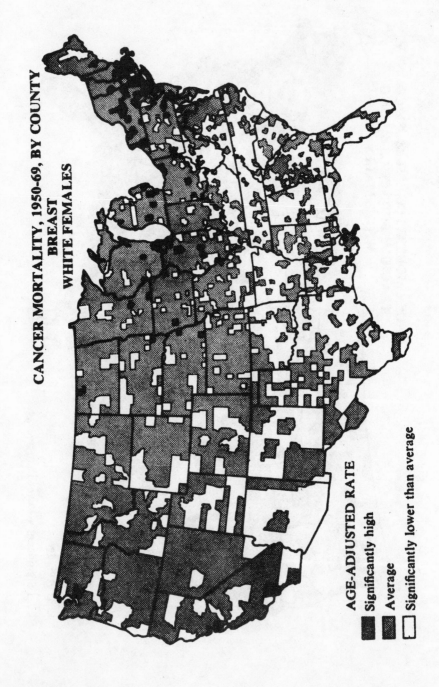

CANCER MORTALITY, 1950-69, BY COUNTY
BREAST
WHITE FEMALES

AGE-ADJUSTED RATE

■ Significantly high

■ Average

□ Significantly lower than average

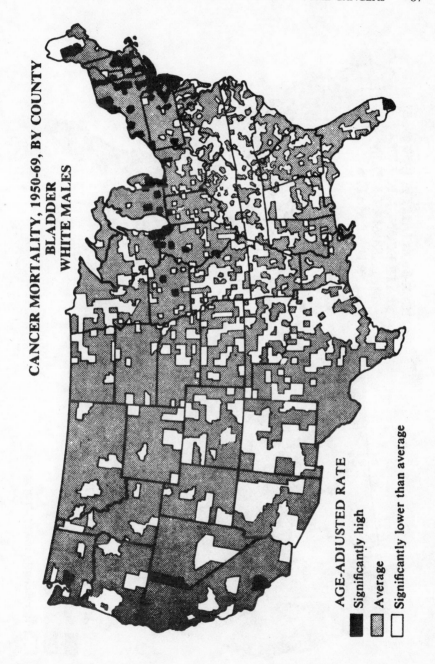

CANCER MORTALITY, 1950-69, BY COUNTY
BLADDER
WHITE MALES

AGE-ADJUSTED RATE

■ Significantly high

▨ Average

□ Significantly lower than average

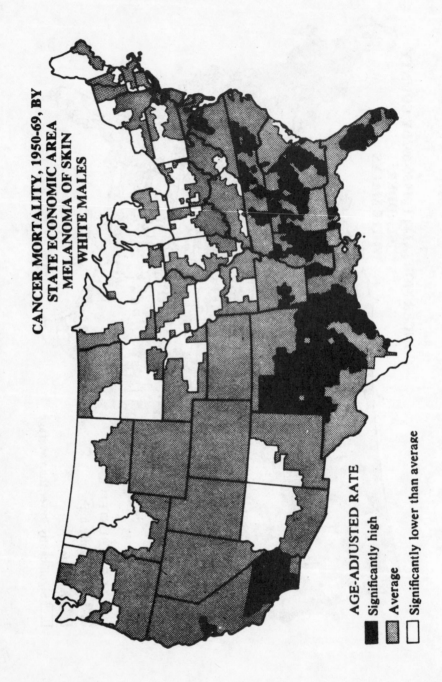

CANCER MORTALITY, 1950-69, BY
STATE ECONOMIC AREA
MELANOMA OF SKIN
WHITE MALES

AGE-ADJUSTED RATE

■ Significantly high

▨ Average

☐ Significantly lower than average

CHAPTER 15

Other Protective Food Factors

So far we have examined several vitamins and minerals for their proven individual roles in protection against cancer. There is no mistake that these individual nutrients are protective. This has been proved by laboratory animal studies where the only variable was that particular pure nutrient, and has been confirmed by epidemiological studies. However, there is more.

Foods contain many hundreds of compounds, and many compounds also have protective roles against cancer. It is important to take advantage of all these compounds by making sure that you eat plenty of fruits and vegetables. It is *then* wise to increase your protection by taking additional amounts of the proven protective nutrients.

I emphasize this dual approach for two reasons. First and most important, it is the only approach that gives optimal protection. Secondly, this approach balances the statements by some scientists who still believe that it hasn't been proven that the individual nutrients are protective—they keep holding out that there may be some other factor(s) in fruits and vegetables that provides the protection.

Unfortunately, these scientists are aware only of the epidemiological studies that indicate fruits and vegetables are protective, and they have a strong but unfounded prejudice against food supplements. These scientists do not seem to be aware of the studies on laboratory animals that prove that individual nutrients are protective. However, they do have a point that there are indeed other compounds that are also protective and we should get ample fruits and vegetables in our diets.

Fruits and Vegetables

A moderate increase in the amount of fruits and vegetables consumed by the "average" person even provides significant protection against tobacco- and alcohol-related cancers such as cancers of the mouth, throat and esophagus.[1]

The point is that it doesn't take that much of an effort to reduce your risk of cancer from even the most potent carcinogens. When the cancer rates for those who eat the recommended amounts are compared to those who eat few fruits and vegetables, typically we see a reduction in risk by one-half, and for some cancers, a 70 percent reduction.[2]

Unfortunately, too few of us eat the recommended five or more servings a day. Several surveys indicate that only about 23 to 25 percent of us do eat the recommended five servings. On the average, we eat only about three-and-a-half servings per day. On any given day, only one in five Americans ate a fibrous or cruciferous vegetable, and only 28 percent ate a fruit or vegetable rich in vitamin C.

When Dr. Gladys Block was at the National Cancer Institute, she led a long-term dietary study of about 11,000 persons. She found that 40 percent of Americans do not eat a single fruit on a typical day, and 20 percent don't eat a single vegetable.[3] Also, half of us don't eat vegetables other than potatoes and salads.

What are some of these protective compounds found in fruits and vegetables? Here are a few of the major food factors of current interest.

LYCOPENE

Lycopene is a carotenoid antioxidant compound that, unlike beta-carotene, does not produce vitamin A in the body. It may be a more powerful antioxidant than beta-carotene, but it may not affect gap-junctional communications. Lycopene has been shown to be an effective protector against cancer.

CANTHAXANTHIN

Canthaxanthin is also a member of the carotenoid family that offers significant protection against cancer.

LUTEIN

Lutein is also a promising antioxidant carotenoid. Lutein gives the red color to tomatoes, red peppers and ruby-red grapefruit, which, of course, are good sources of lutein.

TOCOTRIENOLS

These antioxidants are very similar to the tocopherols, and are members of the vitamin E family. They have also been shown to have protective action against cancer.

GLUCARATE, SULFORAPHANE AND DITHIOLTHIONES

Cruciferous vegetables (broccoli, brussels sprouts, cabbage and cauliflower) contain several compounds that have cancer-preventing properties. These include glucarate, sulforaphane and dithiolthiones. These compounds appear to reduce existing tumors as well. The cruciferous vegetables also contain several isothiocyantes and phenolic-based compounds that may show some anti-cancer activity. Phenethyl isothiocyanate appears to have an effect against lung cancer. You can take advantage of all of these compounds by eating a diverse diet that includes the various cruciferous vegetables.

PYCNOGENOL, QUERCETIN AND RUTIN

Pycnogenol (tm), quercetin and rutin are bioflavonoids that have been shown to inhibit cancer.

EPIGALLOCATECHIN GALLATE

Green tea is being widely researched for its cancer-preventing properties. Considerable evidence is accumulating that the epigallocatechin gallate found in green tea is an antioxidant and very effective in protecting against cancer.

EICOSAPENTAENOIC ACID (EPA) AND GAMMA-LINOLENIC ACID (GLA)

Vegetables contain oils that are rich in polyunsaturated fatty acids which can easily be peroxidized unless we eat sufficient amounts of the antioxidant nutrients. Vegetable oils are generally polyunsaturated fatty acids of the type called "omega-6" fatty acids. There are two other types of polyunsaturated fatty acids that are important to health, too, but most Americans are deficient in them. They are the omega-3 fatty acid, eicosapentaenoic acid (EPA) and the omega-1 fatty acid, gamma-linolenic acid (GLA).

The latter two have been shown to have cancer protection activity, whereas most omega-6 vegetable oils have been shown to have cancer-promoting activity. EPA is found in cold-water fish and GLA is found in evening primrose oil, borage and black-currant oil.

ELLAGIC ACID

Ellagic acid, which is found in fruits and nuts, inhibits cancer and is active against substances that can initiate cancer. Rich sources of ellagic acid include strawberries, raspberries, cranberries, loganberries, cashews, pecans, walnuts, and Brazil nuts. Other significant sources include cherries, oranges, grapes, plums and apples.

GARLIC AND SULFUR NUTRIENTS

Just a reminder that there are several good sulfur-containing nutrients in garlic—ajoenes, diallyl sulfide, dithiins and other thiols—that are protective against cancer.

LIMONENE

Limonene is a terpene found in orange peels that has anti-cancer activity. While this may not be a part of your diet, it may find use as a treatment for cancer in the future.

CONJUGATED LINOLEIC ACID (CLA)

A long-chain fatty acid called conjugated linoleic acid (CLA) is a powerful antioxidant that can quench free radicals.

THE MESSAGE

The message of this chapter is simply "Eat your five servings daily of fruits and vegetables." We still have a lot to learn about their outstanding value in protecting us against cancer. But *also* take the proven nutrients that we have discussed, especially beta-carotene, vitamin A, vitamin C, vitamin E and the trace mineral selenium.

REFERENCES

1. D. M. Winn et al., "Diet in the etiology of oral and pharyngeal cancer among women from the southern United States," *Cancer Research* (March 1984) 44(3):1216–22.
2. Graham A. Colditz et al., "Increased green and yellow vegetable intake and lowered cancer deaths in an elderly population," *American Journal of Clinical Nutrition* (Jan. 1985) 41(1):32–6.
3. Gladys Block, B. Patterson, and A. Subar, "Fruit, vegetables, and cancer prevention: a review of the epidemiological evidence," *Nutrition and Cancer* (1992) 18(1):1–29.

CHAPTER 16

Shark Cartilage Destroys Cancer Tumors

There are always several promising developments ongoing in the science of natural food supplements in preventing or treating cancer. I use measured restraint in reporting these to you, as some will never prove as effective after additional testing as was suggested by preliminary results. On the other hand, if I fail to report a major development to you, I have not provided you with all the knowledge that you need to develop your anti-cancer strategy.

I have been monitoring a development that promises to be the most important health development that I have ever witnessed. Cancer is a horrible disease, and anything that will reduce the awful suffering and premature deaths of hundreds of thousands of cancer victims is the most important health event in the century.

In this case, I decided to delay the publication until clinical results from studies that meet my requirements became available. However, it will be years before several large-scale tests confirm these early clinical trials; since the early trials were designed with significant checks, their results will most likely be reproduced in larger confirmational studies.

I have been discussing the progress of specially processed shark cartilage in preventing tumor growth with Dr. I. William Lane. Dr. Lane received both his B.A. and M.A. in the field of Nutritional Science from Cornell University. He received his Ph.D. in Agricultural Biochemistry and Nutrition from Rutgers University. As a researcher, he studied and worked under two Nobel prize winners, Dr. James B. Sumner (NP-1946) and Dr. Selman A. Waksman (NP-1952).

Dr. Lane applied his research in poultry nutrition in association with Perdue Farms, Inc. and Tyson Food, Inc. Later he became a vice president for W. R. Grace and Company, Inc., heading its Marine Resources Division. This experience in biochemistry and marine science provided Dr. Lane with a special background to pursue his more than ten years of research with shark cartilage.

Serendipitously, Dr. Lane, in the course of his research, found that this specially processed shark cartilage not only halted tumor growth, it also destroyed existing tumors. In 1992, Dr. Lane published a book about his early research and I had the opportunity to interview him for *Whole Foods* magazine.[1] I will share some of that interview with you so that you can hear of this amazing discovery directly from Dr. Lane.

As I mentioned in Chapter 5, cancer is a multi-step process in which cells accumulate multiple genetic alterations as they progress to a more malignant mutation. Although there are many steps, they can be grouped into three distinct phases. My research has concentrated on preventing the first step, while Dr. Lane's research has concentrated on preventing the third step, and more importantly, *eliminating cancer tumors* in advanced cancer patients.

The first step in the process is the damage caused by agents known as carcinogens. Carcinogens can damage critical parts of genes called proto-oncogenes directly or by generating free radicals. Carcinogens may be chemicals, radiation or viruses. Antioxidant nutrients protect against damage that can be caused by carcinogens.

Initiating the development process does not necessarily lead to cancer. This process alone will only produce a series of independent precancerous cells. In order for cancer to develop, the process must be propagated to the point where these precancerous cells will reproduce, associate and develop their own blood supply and defense system. If there is no propagation or if the immune system is activated and destroys these precancerous cells, then cancer will not develop.

The second step in cancer development, called "promotion," allows the precancerous cells to reproduce rapidly and change their membrane surface properties to those characteristic of malignant cells. Anything that promotes cell reproduction decreases the chance that repair enzymes will repair (deactivate) the activated oncogene.

Even with promotion, the proliferating cells will not necessarily develop into cancer. The cell mass must grow large enough to affect body metabolism and start its own blood supply and defense system. This is the third step, called "progression." Progression leads to cancer, including the malignant tumors of carcinoma (consisting largely of epithelial cells) and adenocarcinoma (cancer of a gland), and eventually metastasis (the invasive spreading to other areas).

I am excited about Dr. Lane's *clinical* studies showing that shark cartilage is eliminating tumors in Stages III and IV terminal cancer patients. If additional and larger human clinical trials by others confirm these results, it truly will be the most important health news that I have ever heard.

Conventional therapies try to cure cancer by killing more cancer cells than healthy cells. Dr. Lane found in his search why sharks don't get cancer, that the process that stops the third step in cancer development also can be used to eliminate existing cancers. He was the right man with the right background at the right place at the right time. Later, I'll get to his dramatic clinical studies showing that shark cartilage destroys malignant tumors with great efficiency, but let's start near the beginning.*

PASSWATER: You have found that a specially processed natural food product not only stops tumor growth, but destroys existing tumors. You discuss this in your book which is entitled, *Sharks Don't Get Cancer*. I've never worked with a laboratory room

---

*[The following is reproduced with permission of *Whole Foods* magazine.]

full of sharks—at least not the finned kind. Is your title an exaggeration to make a point, and is it relevant whether or not sharks get cancer?

LANE: "Never" is a slight exaggeration to make an important point. Actually, as we stated in the book, some cancer has been reported in sharks, but fewer than one in a million sharks show cancer—less than 1 percent of the incidence of tumors reported for all other species of fish. What is relevant is that sharks rarely get cancer and that this fact has been tied specifically to their cartilage skeleton and the strong anti-tumor activity of shark cartilage. Sharks have absolutely no bones, but a relatively large amount of cartilage that contains factors which protect against cancer. Six to eight percent of a shark's weight is cartilage, which is about 1,000 times the amount of cartilage found in a calf of the same weight. Also, shark cartilage is slightly different from that of mammals.

PASSWATER: I have also been following the research of Dr. Robert Langer of the Massachusetts Institute of Technology and the preliminary research of Dr. John Prudden, a Harvard-trained physician, showing a factor in cartilage that inhibited tumors.[2-4] What is different about cartilage that would explain why this factor is present in cartilage?

LANE: In 1976, Dr. Robert Langer showed that shark cartilage contained an inhibitor of new blood vessels in tumors. When the body makes new blood vessels, the process is called "neovascularization" or "angiogenesis." Angiogenesis is the term most often used, and it is derived from "angio" meaning "pertaining to blood vessels" and "genesis" meaning "formation of," thus "angiogenesis" merely means the origin and development of blood vessels.

　　Earlier, Dr. Judah Folkman of Harvard had put forth the theory that one could prevent a tumor from exceeding 1 to 2 square millimeters (the size of a pencil point) if a blood network could be prevented from forming.[5] A blood network is needed to feed the tumor and remove waste products. This concept opened up a whole new strategy for controlling cancer and is the approach with which I have been working.

In 1983, Drs. Anna Lee and Robert Langer pinpointed the mechanism to this approach which I had been following. They reported that an extract of shark cartilage inhibited both new blood vessel growth and tumor development.[6] They also showed the inhibitor to be 1,000 times more concentrated in the shark cartilage, when processed to remove the fat as Dr. John Prudden did, is very low in blood vessel inhibiting activity. Rather, bovine cartilage relies primarily on its ability to stimulate the immune system with mucopolysaccharides (glycosaminoglycans, a class of complex carbohydrates) which is a positive, but weak, development, nowhere near the magnitude of importance or effectiveness of antiangiogenesis (preventing blood vessel development).

It was postulated that the logical place to look for such natural inhibitors of angiogenesis would be in tissue not having blood vessels (avascular). The most common avascular tissue is cartilage. The theory being that cartilage is avascular because it contains inhibitors of new vascularization, and that shark cartilage, pound for pound, is by far the most actively antiangiogenic.

PASSWATER: When we last spoke, you mentioned that several antiangiogenic factors have been discovered in cartilage, and that this is a distinct advantage of your whole cartilage food over a purified drug which is a single compound. What type of compounds are these antiangiogenic factors, and how sensitive are they to environmental factors such as processing?

LANE: It is believed that all of the antiangiogenic factors in shark cartilage are proteins. In late 1992, two separate proteins, both with major antiangiogenic properties, have been identified, one by Dr. Robert Langer, and a second by Japanese researchers.[7,8] It is postulated that as many as five separate active antiangiogenic proteins are in shark cartilage. With the whole shark cartilage properly prepared, all work synergistically. Proteins are easily denatured (inactivated) by heat, acids, alcohols, acetones, and many other chemicals. Thus, proper processing to prevent denaturization is most important.

The mucopolysaccharides and their ability to stimulate the

immune system, as found in shark and other cartilage, are important, but I believe that most, if not all, of the activity I am showing comes from the antiangiogenic proteins.

PASSWATER: Shark cartilage keeps a tumor from growing by inhibiting the formation of the new blood vessels that are needed to feed the tumor. How do you explain how shark cartilage destroys existing tumors?

LANE: The blood network of a tumor is fragile. Tumor capillaries are different and may be considered "immature" compared to normal capillaries. Their walls are thinner and decidedly more fragile. Tumor blood vessels are constantly breaking down and being replaced by new vessels. When the existing vessels break down in the presence of antiangiogenesis factors, they are not replaced by new vessels and the section fed by the vessels dies (necrosis). You can see this when such a tumor is cut open. Instead of pinkish tissue, the tissue is gray. Then it decays away and leaves an air-space. I refer to the appearance of air spaces—especially in large breast tumors—-as "the Swiss cheese effect."

PASSWATER: Can you verify and quantify your claim that shark cartilage has more antiangiogenic activity than bovine or other cartilage?

LANE: Yes, the scientific literature documents this fact. Dr. Robert Langer of the Massachusetts Institute of Technology has studied various cartilages and reports in the highly respected peer-reviewed scientific journal *Science* that shark cartilage is 1,000 times more potent in antiangiogenic factor, all of which is in the protein fraction, than bovine or other mammalian cartilage.

PASSWATER: How can we be sure that significant amounts of antiangiogenic factor are in shark cartilage products?

LANE: In the life and death matter of clinical research, we must be certain of the efficacy of the product used. A standard assay method developed by Dr. Judah Folkman of the Harvard Medical School, Dr. Robert Langer of Massachusetts Institute of Technology, and others, called the CAM (short for chick chorioallantoic membrane) assay allows one to measure the angiogenesis inhibiting capability of a product. This assay involves adding the material to be tested to a fertilized chicken egg yolk sac and measuring the amount of new blood vessel development under standardized conditions.

Using the CAM assay one can, and should, control production lots. I used the CAM assay early on in my research to improve production methods. I was able to materially increase inhibition activity using the CAM assay as a guide, and I continue to seek better processing methods constantly.

PASSWATER: Has commercially processed shark cartilage been effective against human cancers?

LANE: Studies with only advanced cases—usually stage III and stage IV terminal patients—with shark cartilage as the only therapy have shown results which are most significant. In eight breast tumor cases where the tumors were all larger than golf balls in size, all eight women were tumor-free or approaching a tumor-free state in eleven weeks. In three other studies on breast cancer, the results have been the same. With 76 cancer cases in the United States, a New Jersey physician has shown all 76 patients responding to the shark cartilage therapy. The shark cartilage therapy works on all solid tumors, but appears to be most effective with breast, liver, brain and esophageal tumors, where major changes within four to six weeks are noticeable. Lung and prostate cancers seem to respond more slowly, and we have seen good responses with pancreatic tumors at very high dosage levels.

PASSWATER: How have these studies demonstrated that it was the shark cartilage and not some residual effect of other treatments that was effective?

LANE: Residual effect is always a possibility; however, in a clinical trial in Cuba on 27 advanced cancer victims, no patient was selected that had not been off other therapies for at least several weeks, and in the three Mexican studies, all patients had been off all other therapies for extended periods. In practice, many patients not in clinical trials do take the shark cartilage along with other therapies like chemotherapy or radiation therapy. No one wants to suggest countermanding a physician's suggestions, but patients want the shark cartilage because they doubt the positive effects of much conventional therapy and have had good reports on the effect of shark cartilage.

PASSWATER: How do we know that the tumors are actually being destroyed?

LANE: In all clinical trials and with all patients of Dr. Martinez in New Jersey, starting-point, mid-point and end-point scans by either MRI (magnetic resonance imaging) or CAT (computer-assisted tomography) are done to follow the progress of tumor tissue death (necrosis). These scans often show the development of air spaces in the tumors as the malignant tissue dies away due to lack of a blood supply as the therapy progresses. Many radiologists who are not used to seeing tumor necrosis in advanced cancer often are puzzled about the appearance of air spaces, and they often suspect abscesses. All that this is, is the Swiss-cheese effect that I mentioned earlier.

PASSWATER: What clinical trials are now under way?

LANE: The clinical trial led by Dr. Martinez is ongoing, as is a 27-patient study in Cuba. I expect another clinical trial to get under way in Cuba that will include breast, uterine/cervical, brain, and esophageal cancer patients, with 30 patients included in each cancer category. In Germany, four patients are being treated with shark cartilage by Dr. Helmut Keller, and in Austria, four patients each with Drs. Steinheller and Werkmann are just starting treatment.

In all of these studies, MRI scans, blood chemistries and photographs will be taken so that publications can be forthcoming. My problem has been the lack of funding for extensive clinical trials, especially in the United States.

PASSWATER: Just how much shark cartilage is required to treat human cancers?

LANE: My first study in Mexico was based on the equivalent of 60 grams of whole shark cartilage per day based on body weight of under–140-pound patients. At this time in trials, we have gone as high as 120 grams daily with advanced cancer cases. An average of 60 to 80 grams daily is generally used, and the success rate with solid tumors has been higher than 80 percent. The shark cartilage is administered orally in juice or buttermilk at the rate of 15 to 20 grams each time, spread throughout the day and taken between meals. In some advanced cases, and in the Cuban study, all is administered rectally at the rate of 15 to 20 grams in four ounces of body-temperature water. These enemas are given four times daily as retention enemas.

After one becomes tumor-free (metastases and all), a preventative dose of 10 to 15 grams daily probably should be used for an extended time, but to date, I have no specific data on this.

PASSWATER: What do we know about the safety of shark cartilage?

LANE: Shark cartilage—like all active materials—must be used properly. Since it inhibits new vascularization, those having suffered a recent coronary occlusion (heart attack), pregnant women and those wanting to conceive, and people recovering from recent surgery should all refrain from use for a logical time period.

We have experienced some stomach upsets, primarily with those on a macrobiotic or vegetarian diet who also respond more slowly. We see some very limited allergic responses, but in general, most people can use shark cartilage with no problems at all.

The cost of the high-dosage therapy will generally be between $2,000 to $3,000 to reach a tumor-free state based on clinical experience covering a period under 16 weeks. This is only a small fraction of the cost of conventional therapy, and, based on the clinical studies conducted so far, the success rate is far superior.

PASSWATER: I remember what happened to the Pacific yews in Oregon when it was found that taxol (tamoxifen), the experimental drug being studied to treat breast cancer, could be extracted from their bark. Will sharks be endangered by our need to cure human cancer?

LANE: About 10 million sharks are caught each year, based on statistics of shark fin usage for the shark-fin soup market. If the heads and backbones, representing most of the cartilage, were kept and used, there would be enough shark cartilage to treat 625,000 cancer patients a year without catching a single additional shark than are caught now. It would just be greater utilization of material now thrown away unused. Hopefully, synthesis of the active components will follow shortly as well.

PASSWATER: My research was presented to the National Cancer Institute in 1978, but it has only been recently that they became interested in it. Didn't you present your research to them also?

LANE: Yes! I did present my research to the National Cancer Institute in 1991. I gave a seminar for Dr. Robert Gallo and thirty of his top research scientists, and they gave me a standing ovation and an immediate offer to collaborate. However, within three months, the offer to work with me was withdrawn and no acceptable excuse was given. I assume it was because there was a resistance to work with a natural product. They have followed my research, however, and it has been been written up in the July 1992 *Journal of the National Cancer Institute*. However, no offer to renew collaboration was ever made to my knowledge, even though I am told that patients phoning the National Cancer Institute and asking about shark cartilage are given encouraging comments in general.

PASSWATER: Did your research lead to any patents?

LANE: On Christmas Eve (December 24, 1991), I was granted United States Patent #5,075,112 covering the use of shark cartilage to inhibit angiogenesis. This patent was fully supported by CAM assay and showing the inhibition of angiogenesis by shark cartilage. A second patent covering the processing techniques used in manufacture has been applied for.

PASSWATER: Dr. Lane, I don't know what to say. This is the most exciting development that I have ever experienced. I encourage everyone to read your book, and we all will be looking for the results from your next round of studies.

At the time of this writing, not only were the cancer patients given a thorough before and after documentation study, the patients' progress was also monitored by the CBS television show "60 Minutes." Reporter Mike Wallace interviewed on videotape patients entering the clinical study in Cuba and then he interviewed them after treatment in January 1993. The "60 Minutes" staff scrutinized the process and researchers very thoroughly and presented their findings in mid-February 1993.

The "60 Minutes" program concluded, "Shark cartilage therapy was a promising treatment." Mike Wallace also stated that "60 Minutes" would be following these patients, as well as other studies, closely.

You the reader, will have the advantage of checking into additional follow-up studies. However, if I hadn't told you about it here, you might never have heard of this unlikely destroyer of cancer tumors. Let us all hope that the medical establishment will allow the tests to continue and will give it a fair deal. After all, if a natural product is successful, a lot of people in the research community will have to find other research projects and many physicians who treat cancer with competing methods will lose a large source of income. This should be an interesting course of events to follow.

In the meantime, I pray that it eliminates a lot of needless suffering.

REFERENCES

1. I. William Lane and Linda Comac, *Sharks Don't Get Cancer*, (Garden City, New York: Avery, 1992).
2. Robert Langer et al., "Isolation of a cartilage factor that inhibits tumor neovascularization," *Science* (1976) 193:70–2.
3. Anne Lee and Robert Langer, "Shark cartilage contains inhibitors of tumor angiogenesis," *Science* (1983) 221:1185–7.
4. John F. Prudden, "The treatment of human cancer with agents prepared from bovine cartilage," *Journal of Biological Response Modifiers* (1985) 4:551–84.
5. Judah Folkman, "Tumor angiogenesis: Therapeutic implications," *New England Journal of Medicine* (1971) 285:1182–6.
6. Anne Lee and Robert Langer, "Shark cartilage contains inhibitors of tumor angiogenesis," *Science* (1983) 221:1185–7.
7. Marsha A. Moses, Judith Sudhalter, and Robert Langer, "Identification of an inhibitor of neovascularization from cartilage," *Science* (1990) 248:1408–10.
8. H. Oihawa et al., "A novel angiogenic inhibitor derived from Japanese shark cartilage," *Cancer Letters* (1990) 51:181–6.

CHAPTER 17

Other Therapies and Basic Strategy

Cancer therapies are constantly improving. In fact, I am hopeful that shark cartilage and its further refinements will be a major advance, but only time will tell. The conventional therapies are edging ahead little by little, but major advances come from out of the blue. What is written today is soon obsolete. What I hope to offer here is a basic strategy to follow regardless of whether the year is 1994 or 2094, along with a discussion of some so-called alternative therapies.

As a scientist, I can only base my opinions and advice on published clinical studies and the experience that I have had in following patients who have written to me after following my suggestions given in the earlier *Cancer and Its Nutritional Therapies*. Thousands have written to me, expressing their opinion that my advice has saved their lives and that they have overcome their cancers. We don't know for a fact that my advice had anything to do with their recoveries, but I appreciate their kind letters and occasional "God Blesses."

My advice to cancer patients is simple: **Get your immune system into peak shape!** Your basic strategy should be similar to that of the fire service. Firefighters don't waste time chasing a fire. They systematically limit the damage and then destroy the fire. A cancer tumor rarely kills. It's the spread of cancers to vital organs and the depression of the immune system that allows other diseases to develop that usually are the killers.

The priorities of the fire department are in this order: rescue, prevent spread to other buildings, confinement, extinguishment. With cancer, your first priority is to do what you must to stay alive long enough for the treatment to take effect.

Your second priority is to keep the cancer from spreading (metastasizing). If surgery is planned, the procedure could let cancer cells into the bloodstream that could result in metastasis. Even biopsies can (although rarely) spread cancer cells. Secondary cancers that later develop along the biopsy needle's tracks have been observed, but not frequently.

Your strategy here is to prime up your immune system as quickly as possible, even before any biopsy or surgery, if possible. Your tactics are to take the nutrients as discussed in earlier chapters. This will be discussed in more detail under the specific recommendations that follow.

Your next priority is the same as the second, in that you want to isolate any existing cancer so that treatment will be effective and there will be no metastases. Your tactics are to continue the stimulation of your immune system during any treatment that you elect. **Keep in mind that surgery, chemotherapy and radiation all dramatically impair the immune system, and if you are to benefit from their effect, you must strengthen your immune system before, during and after treatment!**

Only now are you ready to go after cancer tumors themselves. There are many treatments to choose from, but even without treatments, some cancers "spontaneously" disappear. This is due to the immune system finally being restored to peak efficiency and attacking the tumor. Though this is sometimes sufficient in itself, you can't afford the risk of hoping that it will work for you. You can now go for the destruction of the tumor itself, which makes the chances of your immune system finishing the job much greater.

These are the steps that I recommend to my friends and family:

1. Seek out the *best* treatment available for your particular cancer. Call the National Cancer Institute for a referral to the medical center that is at the forefront in treating that particular cancer. Do not seek an *experimental* treatment unless there is no alternative. The National Cancer Institute is in Bethesda, Maryland, and they operate the Cancer Information Service, telephone number 1-800-4-CAN-CER. Later in this chapter, I will give you some alternative sources.

    No one medical center is at the forefront for all cancers. Being a year or two behind the forefront might mean the difference between you surviving or not.

2. Go to that center for a second opinion. Do they have a treatment there that is proven to be better than the treatment being offered at your local center, or can you get appropriate treatment in your local medical center?

3. Are you willing to give it your best shot or do you choose to undergo their second choice of treatment? It's your life, but others love you. It sometimes is a tough decision, but you must give whatever treatment you choose your total effort.

4. Begin *immediately* to strengthen your immune system by taking the nutrients that were discussed earlier in this book. If you are reading this book for its advice on treating cancer, you probably skipped over the chapters on prevention of cancer. The nutrients that are protective against cancer also build the immune system to help your body overcome cancer. Go back and read the chapters on prevention.

5. After you have received the best conventional therapy possible, hopefully you are cured. If for some reason, such as that the cancer was too advanced for the treatment, or an effective treatment has not yet been developed for your particular cancer, then you may wish to try an "alternative" treatment. In any case do not give up hope.

Orthodoxy

As pointed out near the beginning of this book, cancer is big business and the powerful politics of cancer are geared to benefit the economics of the controlling factors—the orthodoxy who treat and sell supplies to those who treat by surgery, chemotherapy or radiation. This is not to say that these are evil forces—just economic forces. The economics of the situation tend to discourage changes to the system that don't benefit the system.

With this said, however, we must put our trust with this imperfect system as it appears to be the best system we have at this writing. However, we can improve the system. We must force the orthodoxy to open their eyes and minds by exposing them to facts that they may be overlooking.

The orthodoxy is making progress, although it is very slow. As in the case of shark cartilage, as facts become available, they should be brought to the orthodoxy's attention. The usual response is denial, followed by personal attacks on the originators of new ideas. As evidence accumulates, others will join in the research, and finally after years of violent "debate," the evidence will be examined on its own merits. Then, and only then, we will have an answer.

My point is that current wisdom can lead to the cure of only half of the cancer cases. The innovation that will boost this cure rate dramatically most likely will come from a new direction. Will it be shark cartilage? Will it be a new idea? Will it be an old "unproven" treatment that has not yet been given proper scrutiny?

In the meantime, we have to go with what little evidence we have that we can trust. Therefore, even though some of the orthodox treatments are worse than the disease, I recommend starting with the orthodoxy. I do not recommend starting with "alternative" methods, until and unless evidence can be presented that would make that a wise choice. Therein lies a problem. How do supporters of new therapies pay for the expense of developing appropriate studies unless they are funded by others, and such funds-granting organizations are "controlled" by those that economically benefit from the status quo. This is a Catch-22 situation, but let's take a look at the politics so that you can understand the difference between the "orthodox" and the "alternative" approaches.

Dr. Ralph W. Moss describes the problem in his book, *The Cancer Industry* (Paragon House, 1989). Dr. Moss was once an "insider" in the cancer industry. He was a researcher at the Memorial Sloan-Kettering Cancer Center who states that his group was finding positive results from the drug laetrile at a time when the orthodoxy was attempting to discredit it. In his book, Dr. Moss describes the huge profits that are made within the existing treatment approaches. He believes that research institutions, hospitals, medical associations, government agencies, foundations, and large corporations make great efforts to thwart research and testing of alternative, nontoxic therapies.

Dr. Moss stops short of stating that he believes that it is a conscious conspiracy, but he feels that in pursuing their goal of amassing power, profit or prestige that all are, in effect, united against any innovation that could upset the status quo. Dr. Moss supports his opinion with a vast arsenal of facts that make one's mind spin.

You can see that there is at least the potential for politics to influence science. And, of course, there is always a second point of view. Orthodoxy has had its fill of cancer hoaxes and scams knowingly perpetuated by medical quacks—usually physicians. Physicians are dealing with life and death matters, and they must "first do no harm." They must be conservative and choose "accepted," although not necessarily proven, treatments.

But what happens when a physician develops a new treatment that he or she honestly believes is better, and has had good success with, but does not have the funds, time or inclination to conduct the double-blind, placebo-controlled, crossover, clinical studies required for FDA approval? **These studies cost an average of $231 million (1990 dollars) and take 12 years to win approval, according to a Tufts University study.** Do some of these alternative therapies have something to offer the cancer patient who has not been helped by orthodox treatment?

Alternative Therapies

In 1986, several members of the U.S. Congress asked this very same question after hearings in which many former cancer patients testified to the benefits of various alternative therapies. More than 40 members of Congress requested that the U.S. Office of Technology Assessment (OTA) study the available evidence.

When the 500-page study was presented to Congress, Roger C. Herdman, Assistant Director of the OTA's Health and Sciences Division, said that "We didn't find any miraculous cures, and there was a paucity of scientific evidence—either pro or con—for alternative cancer treatments. But, it's a big enough issue for the federal government to do more work and to evaluate these treatments where suggestive evidence can be produced and to show that it's justified."

So we waited for four years for an informed report, and the report says that what is needed is further study.[1]

It is not an easy task. There are many errors, omissions and half-truths in the OTA report, but the OTA is correct in saying that there is a paucity of information both pro and con on alternative therapies. However, this hasn't stopped either side from making strong and emotional claims. An article by Dr. Robert Houston of New York City discusses the many errors.[2]

Dr. Linus Pauling is correct in pointing out how the Mayo Clinic's study was not related to the treatment that Dr. Cameron and he recommend (see Chapter 8). Dr. Moss is correct in pointing out that the Memorial Sloan-Kettering report was a hatchet job on laetrile. But the fact that the attempts of the orthodoxy to dismiss an alternative therapy merely out of prejudice have been shown to be incorrect does not necessarily mean that the alternative therapies do indeed work.

I will attempt to give you a little background and my personal—but necessarily incomplete—opinion on a few of the most promising alternative therapies. Some are nutritional therapies, others are not. Hopefully, more information will become available on these therapies after this writing, so I will give you sources for obtaining current information.

SHARK CARTILAGE

Shark cartilage destroys tumors by preventing the tumors from developing and maintaining their blood supplies. This therapy can be given in conjunction with conventional treatments, and was the subject of the preceding chapter. At this writing, this looks as if it's going to be the most promising weapon against cancer tumors developed yet, and may be the "outside factor" that increases cancer cure rate from 50 percent to 80-90 percent.

IMMUNO-AUGMENTATIVE THERAPY

Any agent that stimulates the immune system will benefit cancer patients. As mentioned throughout this book, the antioxidant nutrients are effective immune system boosters. However, certain agents could possibly be even more effective. One of the most widely known methods, according to the OAT, is the Immuno-Augmentative Therapy (IAT).

A vaccine developed by Dr. Lawrence Burton is claimed to have extended the lives of many patients and to have made a number free of cancer. The vaccine is composed of processed blood products. As this vaccine involves daily, lifelong injections, Dr. Burton's patients are understandably very eager to testify on behalf of Dr. Burton.

Dr. Burton, a biologist, teamed with Dr. Frank Friedman to investigate two cancer-inhibiting factors. These investigators were Senior Associates in the Hodgkins' Disease Research Laboratory of St. Vincent's Hospital in New York City. Dr. Burton and his colleagues published nearly twenty scientific papers on cancer, with more than five on these cancer-inhibiting factors.[3-7]

The researchers named these two cancer-inhibiting factors "V" and "I." They claimed that injection of these factors eliminated signs of cancer in 26 of 50 mice with cancer. All of the treated group lived longer than the controls.

In another study, 37 of 68 mice with cancer survived 131 days after treatment without any signs of cancer, compared to 12 days for the untreated controls. (Mice normally live from 2 to 2.5 years in laboratory conditions, but it is unclear as to how old the mice were at the time of the treatment.)

At an American Cancer Society seminar for science writers in the mid-1960s, Dr. Burton demonstrated that the injections made solid tumors in mice disappear in one hour. He was accused of fraud by either switching mice or "massaging the tumor until it somehow liquified"! and was extracted with a needle.

Dr. Burton attempted to get Investigational New Drug status with the Food and Drug Administration (FDA), but this process was halted by the FDA due to "inadequate information." Dr. Burton then moved to Freeport, Grand Bahamas to continue his experimental investigations.

As of the 1980s, the experimental treatment utilized four components of the immune system that are extracted from blood. Three components—deblocking protein (DP), tumor antibody 1 (TA1) and tumor antibody 2 (TA2)—are extracted from the blood of healthy donors. The fourth factor, tumor complement (TC), is extracted from blood clots of persons who have cancer.

One of the concerns of the orthodoxy is the possible transmission of other diseases via these blood extractions. However, terminally ill cancer patients do not seem to see that as a major concern.

It seems unlikely that this man with a good scientific background would attempt fraud that would surely be detected; he would know that his results could not be duplicated by others. However, I am not aware of any legitimate attempts to duplicate his research. Dr. Burton appears to have become disenchanted with the orthodoxy because of their unwillingness to follow his findings. They merely scoffed and said, without studying the findings, that the process couldn't work. Therefore, Dr. Burton never again attempted to publish his findings or to teach others how to properly prepare the four blood fractions for his vaccine.

On the one hand, I don't see a dramatic number of persons miraculously cured of cancer. But many respected holistic physicians sent patients to Dr. Burton and believe that the patients were helped. One researcher who studied 50 consecutive patients treated by Dr. Burton estimated that they averaged a survival *at least double* that provided by conventional therapy. Several are still alive and some have met the criteria for being "cured."

As the OTA report indicated, more research is needed. But who is going to step forward and do it? The controversy surrounding IAT will keep capable persons away because they could lose scientific respectability if they became involved. There are few scientists willing to risk their future in this direction, even though it could lead to great discoveries. There aren't many heroes out there, but at least you should know about this experimental treatment.

ANTINEOPLASTONS

Antineoplastons are compounds naturally produced in the body that have antitumor activity. Antineoplastons were discovered by Dr. Stanislaw R. Burzynski in Poland in 1967.[8] Dr. Burzynski now treats cancer patients at the Burzynski Research Institute in Houston with four antineoplastons called A2, A5, A10 and AS2-1. He claims that these nontoxic antineoplastons have caused tumor shrinkage in a number of difficult cases which were not aided by conventional therapies.[8-11]

These antineoplastons are normally found in the blood and urine of healthy persons, but are not present or are present in low amounts in cancer patients. Researchers at the Medical College of Georgia have confirmed that antineoplaston A10 delays or inhibits breast tumors in mice and rats.[12] Also, researchers in Japan have confirmed that antineoplaston A10 reduces breast cancer tumors and lung cancer tumors.[13, 14]

On January 6, 1992, the National Cancer Institute announced that it had "reviewed seven cases of primary brain tumors that were treated by Dr. Burzynski with antineoplastons A10 and AS2-1 and concluded that antitumor responses occurred."

So, you ask, why is this an alternative therapy? Doesn't it sound like orthodoxy research? The problem is that Dr. Burzynski holds the patents on the antineoplaston preparations and not a drug company, university or government. In 1983, the FDA tried to close the Burzynski Research Institute down, but could only prevent the transportation of the antineoplastons across state borders. In 1987, a large

insurance company brought suit against Dr. Burzynski for civil racke-
teering. It was dismissed in 1992. But, in 1992, the Texas Attorney
General attempted to stop all distribution of antineoplastons.

Also in 1992, Dr. Saul Green (Ph.D.) attacked Dr. Burzynski
(M.D., Ph.D.) in the *Journal of the American Medical Association,*
claiming that Dr. Burzynski did not have a Ph.D. (You don't need
a Ph.D. to do research.) Dr. Burzynski does have a sworn statement
from Professor Zdzislaw Kleinrok, president of the Medical Academy of Poland, confirming his Ph.D. in biochemistry was awarded
on October 16, 1968.

This is what happens when you come close to curing cancer, even
if you are a respected scientist and your research is confirmed by
other scientists and published in the peer-reviewed scientific literature.

LAETRILE

I have no new information on laetrile (amygdalin, B-17) since the
last edition of *Cancer and Its Nutritional Therapies* in 1983. You
would think that if there were miracle cures being accomplished
that there would be studies published somewhere. But what journal
would be brave enough to risk losing advertisements and readers
if it did publish on laetrile? After all, the laetrile debates and the
freedom of choice movements were the most emotional issues in
health care in the 1970s.

As I mentioned earlier, Dr. Ralph W. Moss did find positive
results with laetrile in his preliminary studies at Memorial Sloan-
Kettering Cancer Center in New York City. Since he did not go
along with the Center's "hatchet-job" on laetrile, he was dismissed.

Even the OTA reported that earlier work at Memorial Sloan-
Kettering Cancer Center by Dr. Kanematsu Sugiura "did show
inhibition of lung metastases."[1] Even though Dr. Sugiura found
that laetrile stopped metastases (21 percent of mice receiving laetrile
had metastases compared to 90 percent in the control mice) and
inhibited the growth of small tumors in three animal species, other
researchers at Memorial Sloan-Kettering claimed that they could
not reproduce Dr. Sugiura's results.[15]

In earlier editions of *Cancer and Its Nutritional Therapies,* I described the experimental flaws of the Memorial Sloan-Kettering research in the way that the mice were intermingled and given injections based on ear-notch identification. Try this sometime. Would you believe that laboratory animal technicians are perfect in picking out which animals are to be given which shots every day without fail? Can you imagine what happens to ear notches in cages of fighting mice over a long period of time? Yes, the mice did get mixed up because the researchers reported that 40 percent of those receiving saline solution as the placebo were cured of cancer. Do you think that salt water can cure cancer? There was little difference between the salt-water-treated and laetrile-treated groups of mice simply because the technicians got the mice mixed up when administering their daily shots.

The Mayo Clinic tried a clinical trial of laetrile given under the conditions used by its proponents, but found no benefit.[16] The laetrile proponents claimed that the so-called laetrile used by the Mayo Clinic was actually a degraded product.

The Mayo Clinic researchers warned in their summary that some patients showed symptoms of cyanide toxicity or had blood cyanide levels approaching the lethal range, but in the body of the report, they said that "most of these reactions were either mild and transient or . . . possibly not drug-related."[16] What actually happened is that one of the three patients having high cyanide levels also ate large amounts of raw almonds, while the other two patients took double the dosage of laetrile. As few as 12 raw apricot kernels can be dangerous, and even fewer under certain circumstances.

Thus, laetrile may have some merit—not as yet verified—and it may have toxicity if improperly administered. Again, we must wait for a calmer political climate to investigate laetrile. In the 1970s, I spoke with many physicians and patients alike who believed that laetrile therapy produced a noticeable improvement in their cancers. It seemed that physicians were under the impression that maybe 20 to 30 percent of their patients given laetrile dramatically improved or went into remission.

Was it a type of placebo effect or the result of the vitamin therapy simultaneously administered? Who knows? But, since I have not had a cancer patient recently tell me that he or she believed that laetrile had cured their cancer, I do not put laetrile on the recommended list at this time. The burden of the proof lies with the promotors of the therapy. We will probably see another cancer therapy, such as shark cartilage, become prominent before laetrile can be scientifically and impassionately investigated.

MACROBIOTICS

I am often asked about using a macrobiotic diet with cancer therapies. I do recommend eating lots of fruits and vegetables and their juices. There is no harm and maybe benefit in becoming a vegetarian, if you also take the nutrients recommended in the earlier chapters. But the macrobiotic diet as it is practiced in its strictest form seems counterproductive to me. While it is not a "rice diet," nonetheless, it lacks sufficient variety; its rules are too limited to allow normal "vegetarian" selections. It does contain fish, which also helps to distinguish it from a true vegetarian diet.

Yes, there are a few people going around claiming that the macrobiotic diet cured them of cancer and maybe it did. But, in cases where macrobiotics seem to work, the specific circumstances may be too individual to allow it to work in the majority of persons.

I know of no properly conducted clinical trials using the macrobiotic diet, so my observations are strictly opinion. I have witnessed no one being cured by the macrobiotic diet, and I have seen cancer patients on macrobiotic diets fail quickly. However, this is anecdotal and has no scientific meaning. I am also aware of Michio Kushi's teaching and six case histories published by Dr. Vivien Newbold in the *Townsend Letter for Doctors*.[17] But my question remains, how can you predict who will benefit from the macrobiotic diet and who will not? Certainly more research is warranted.

It appears as if there is a problem with the macrobiotic diet in treating cancer in that many of the essential nutrients discussed in earlier chapters are in low supply in the macrobiotic diet. This is opposite of that of a vegetarian diet, which is rich in the antioxidant nutrients.

Macrobiotics (meaning "maximum life") is a strict diet, lifestyle and philosophy. It varies from the traditional Japanese diet and vegetarianism in many ways. The diet is based on "yin" foods grown in hot climates or that have a high acid content or are high in water content, and "yang" foods, which are grown in cold climates or are alkaline or dry.

The macrobiotic diet is 50 to 60 percent whole grains, 25 to 30 percent vegetables, 5 to 10 percent beans, 10 percent seeds, nuts, fruit and fish, and 5 percent soup. It is low in vitamins A, B12 and C, plus calcium. It is also low in calories, which cancer patients need because of their poor appetites. They also need nutrient-dense foods that don't stress the digestive system.

However, a balanced, *moderate* macrobiotic diet with supplements would seem to be protective and offer many of the advantages of vegetarianism.

Gerson Diet

Dr. Max Gerson developed a low-sodium, high-water diet that has several advantages for some.[18, 19] Because it has been around for the longest time, it has been widely attacked by the medical establishment. Orthodoxy is concerned because many people opt for the Gerson diet *instead of* conventional therapy.

I agree that the first choice should be conventional therapy, at least until we have evidence otherwise. But what is wrong with a high fruit and vegetable diet, ample grains, potassium and iodine supplements? The Gerson diet calls for over a dozen glasses of fresh vegetable and fruit juices daily, and a daily vegetable soup. The therapy also includes coffee enemas every three or four hours, which orthodoxy now says is quackery, even though they were a part of their standard *Merck Manual* until 1972. The Gerson diet no longer includes liver juice, due to contamination of commercially available livers. That's a shame, because liver juice would be full of many very useful nutrients.

Krebiozen

This is the first controversy that I remember. While in college in the 1950s, I occasionally found time to read about the FDA efforts to discredit this therapy. I remember reading that the FDA analyzed the material and found that it contained little more than water. This is when I first learned of the scientific limitations of the FDA. I was already using scientific instruments that had the ability to measure compounds in the parts-per-trillion range, and finding compounds in this range that had dramatic biological activity, while the FDA was using techniques that measured little more than parts per thousands, and they were claiming that there could be no activity.

Krebiozen was developed by a scientist with outstanding credentials and regard in the chemical community, Dr. Andrew Ivy. Krebiozen was an extract made from the blood of horses infected with "lumpy jaw disease." This extract probably was an immune enhancer, even though Dr. Ivy considered it an "anti toxin." The orthodoxy drove Dr. Ivy to disgrace and poverty, and krebiozen is not available at this time.

Then why do I bother to mention it? Because at this writing, efforts are being made to re-open the research on Krebiozen and it may become available again in the 1990s. For anyone seeking additional information, contact Herb Bailey, author of the original Krebiozen book, at P. O. Box 636, Sandy Hook, CT 06482.

HOXSEY

If you are seeking an alternative cancer therapy, you will undoubtedly hear of the Hoxsey therapy. It has claimed an 80 percent cure rate and is based on herbs. This is another emotional issue in which there is little, if any, supporting evidence. The OTA report acknowledges that "more recent literature leaves no doubt that Hoxsey's formula . . . does indeed contain many plant substances of *marked therapeutic activity*."[1] A good discussion of the ingredient herbs and their actions is given in Dr. Moss' more recent book, *Cancer Therapy*.[20]

Research is definitely needed to find optimal dosages for various tumors to see what part, if any, these herbs may play in treating cancer.

BREWER HIGH-pH THERAPY

Here is a therapy that I have had to abandon because my colleague Dr. Keith Brewer passed away at the age of 92, and I just can't find enough time to pursue all of my scientific leads. Hopefully, shark cartilage therapy and/or other very promising therapies will negate the need for me to pick up this old trail that Dr. Brewer and I started in 1973. I include it here only for the chance that it might attract the attention of other researchers or at least give them a new idea.

This experimental approach utilizes the element rubidium, a member of the potassium family, which is not known to be essential to humans at this time. Rubidium, like all minerals, can be toxic at high doses. Do not experiment with this on your own.

Rubidium may have a role in mineral transport across defective cell membranes, as are present in cancer cells. Like lithium, which seems to have a role as a mineral transporter across defective membranes in depressed persons, rubidium may have a similar role but in a different membrane defect, one that occurs with cancer.

Our research showed that rubidium decreased the number of tumors and average tumor weight in laboratory animals fed carcinogens or receiving transplanted tumors.[21] This was confirmed by researchers at American University.[22]

Tumors were transplanted into the abdomen of mice and allowed to grow for eight days. The mice were then divided into two groups. The control group was continued on conventional mouse chow. The test group, in addition to the mouse chow, was force-fed 1.1 milligrams per day of rubidium carbonate dissolved in distilled water. At the end of 13 more days, the tumors in the control mice had grown to a very large size; both groups of mice were sacrificed. The tumors were then removed and weighed. The tumors in the rubidium-treated animals weighed only one-eleventh the weight of the tumors in the untreated mice. In addition, the treated animals showed no adverse effects from the cancers. The probability that this marked difference in tumor size could have come about by pure chance is exceedingly small.

Rubidium may reduce the amount of glucose carried into cancer cells by potassium, by a process in which rubidium replaces potassium. Rubidium is above potassium in the Hofmeister electromotive series (4.16 vs. 4.318 v) and is more readily transported into the cell, while at the same time rubidium carries fewer molecules into the cell with it in piggyback fashion than does potassium.

Regardless of the postulated mechanism, it is important for researchers to take note of the reduced numbers of tumors and reduced tumor weights in animals fed rubidium. It is also interesting to know that people inhabiting countries with low cancer rates also tend to have higher rubidium levels in their diets.[23] In the U.S., vegetables and fruits typically contain 35 parts per million of rubidium. We do not know what the optimal dietary amount would be if rubidium does prove to play a vital role in health.

Scientists interested in our research on the possible role of rubidium and tumor inhibition can contact me for the specifics.

More Information

We learn a little more about cancer therapy every day. On some days, there are major advances. How do you find the latest information? I have already given you the address and telephone number for the Cancer Information Office of the National Cancer Institute. Use them! Now I will give you several sources of both "balanced-approach" information and "alternative therapy" information.

Through these sources you can learn of the latest advances of Dr. Hans Nieper of Germany, Dr. Emanuel Revici, Dr. Virginia Livingston, and their successors, and the latest advice of Dr. Ralph Moss. You can obtain information to evaluate BCG, hydrazine sulfate, heat treatment, and dozens of other promising (but unproven) therapies.

Dr. Ralph Moss writes the *Cancer Chronicles* newsletter for People Against Cancer of Otho, Iowa. And Frank Wiewel consults on the telephone with sustaining members of that nonprofit organization.

CANHELP is a service that helps people with cancer find the best treatments, both within and outside conventional practice. For a basic fee of $400 (1993), Patrick M. McGrady, Jr. will consult with you by telephone and send you a customized computer search of the worldwide medical literature.

Here are other important addresses:

Arlin J. Brown Cancer Information Center
P.O. Box 251
Ft. Belvoir, VA 22060
telephone 703-451-8638

Breast Cancer Advisory Center
P.O. Box 224
Kensington, MD 20895
telephone 301-718-7293, fax 301-949-1132

Cancer Control Society
2043 N. Berendo St.
Los Angeles, CA 90027
213-663-7801

Cancer Information Service
Boy Scout Bldg., Rm. 340
Bethesda, MD 20892
800-4-CANCER

CANHELP
311 Paradise Bay Road
Port Ludlow, WA 98365
Send an SASE for a brochure.
206-437-2291

Committee for Freedom of Choice in Medicine
1180 Walnut Ave.
Chula Vista, CA 92011
800-227-4473 or 619-428-8200

Gerson Institute
P.O. Box 430
Bonita, CA 91908
619-472-7450, fax 619-267-6441

International Academy of Holistic Health & Medicine
218 Avenue B
Redondo Beach, CA 90277
310-540-0564

International Academy of Nutrition and Preventive Medicine
P.O. Box 18433
Asheville, NC 28814
704-258-3243, fax 704-251-9206

International Association of Cancer Victors
7740 W. Manchester Ave., #10
Playa del Rey, CA 90293
Send an SASE for a free information packet.
213-822-5032, fax 213-822-5132

People Against Cancer
Box 10
Otho, IA 50569
515-972-4444, fax 515-972-4415

REFERENCES

1. U.S. Congress, Office of Technology Assessment (OTA), "Unconventional cancer treatments," Washington, D.C.: US Government Printing Office, 1990.
2. Robert G. Houston, "Misinformation from OTA on unconventional cancer treatments," *Townsend Letter for Doctors* (Oct. 1990) 676-85.
3. Lawrence Burton, et al., "Isolation of two oncolytic fractions from mouse leukemic tissue," Proceedings of the American Association of Cancer Research (1962) 3:308.
4. Frank Friedman, et al., "The extraction and refinement of two refined antitumor substances," *Transactions of the New York Academy of Science* Ser. II (1962) 25:29-32.
5. Lawrence Burton, et al., "Methods for the determination and alteration of titers of a complex of factors present in blood of neoplastic mice," *Trans. N. Y. Acad. Sci. Ser. II* (1962) 225:33-8.
6. Robert Kassel, et al., "Synergistic action of two refined leukemic tissue extracts in oncolysis of spontaneous tumors," *Trans. N. Y. Acad. Sci. Ser. II* (1962) 25:39-44.
7. Frank Friedman, et al., "Necrosis liquefaction and absorption of C3H mammary tumors resulting from injection of extracts from tumor tissue," *Proceed. Amer. Assoc. Cancer Res.* (1965) 6:20 (Abst. 78).
8. Stanislaw R. Burzynski, "Antineoplastons: History of the research," *Drugs Under Experimental and Clinical Research* (1986) 12S:1-9.

9. Stanislaw R. Burzynski, et al.,"Toxicology studies on antineoplastons," *Drugs Exp. Clin. Res.* (1986) 12S:17-35, 47-55.

10. Stanislaw R. Burzynski and E. Kubove, "Initial clinical study with antineoplaston A2 injections in cancer patients with five year follow-up," *Drugs Exp. Clin. Res.* (1987) 13S:1-12.

11. Stanislaw R. Burzynski, et al., "Phase I clinical studies on antineoplaston A5 injections," *Drugs Exp. Clin. Res.* (1987) 13S:37-43.

12. L. B. Hendry and T. G. Muldoon, "Actions of an endogenous antitumorgenic agent on mammary tumor development and modeling analysis of its capacity for interacting with DNA," *Journal of Steroid Biochemistry and Molecular Biology* (1988) 30:325-8.

13. N. Eriguchi, et al., "Chemopreventive effect of antineoplaston A10 on urethane-induced pulmonary neoplasm in mice," *J. of Japan Soc. Cancer Ther.* (1988) 23:1560-5.

14. K. Hasimoto, et al., "The anticancer effect of antineoplaston A10 on human breast cancer serially transplanted to athymic mice," *J. Japan Soc. Cancer Ther.* (1990) 25:1-5.

15. C. C. Stock, et al., "Antitumor effects of amygdalin in spontaneous animal tumor systems," *Journal of Surgical Oncology* (1978) 10:89-123.

16. C. G. Moertel, et al., "A clinical trial of amygdalin (Laetrile) in the treatment of human cancer," *New England Journal of Medicine* (1982) 306:201-6.

17. Vivien Newbold, "Complete remission of advanced medically incurable cancer in six patients following a macrobiotic approach to healing," *Townsend Letter for Doctors* (Oct. 1990) 628-42.

18. Max Gerson, "Effects of a combined dietary regimen on patients with malignant tumors," *Experimental Medicine and Surgery* (1949) 7:299-317.

19. Max Gerson, "The cure of advanced cancer by diet therapy: a summary of 30 years of clinical experimentation," *Physiological Chemistry and Physics* (1978) 10:449-64.

20. Ralph W. Moss, *Cancer Therapy* (New York: Equinox Press, 1992).

21. A. Keith Brewer and Richard A. Passwater, *American Laboratory* (1976) 8(4):80.

22. A. Keith Brewer, et al., *Cytobios* (1979) 24:99-101.

23. D. H. Calloway, et al., *Ecol, Food & Nutr.* (1974) 3:203.

24. A. Keith Brewer, U. S. Patent 3,470,373

25. S. L. Adelman, et al., *Nature* (1967) 213:718.

26. A. Keith Brewer and Richard A. Passwater, *Amer. Lab.* (1976) 8(4):39-47.

27. Otto Warburg, "The prime cause and prevention of cancer," (Wurzburg, Germany: Konrad Kriltsch, 1969), 1-16.

CHAPTER 18

Lung Cancer
Facts and Hints

Lung cancer is the easiest of all cancers to prevent, even though it is the cancer that is most rapidly increasing in incidence among women. Lung cancer used to be the number-one cancer just in men, but now it has overtaken breast cancer to become the number-one cancer in women as well.

In the late 1980s, smoking was believed to be the cause of over 130,000 lung cancer deaths in the United States. It was also estimated that secondhand smoke was the cause of 2,500 to 8,500 lung cancer deaths. Radon (a radioactive gas found underground and in water) was said to have caused somewhere between 5,000 and 20,000 lung cancer deaths, with the "typical" estimate given of approximately 13,000. Asbestos was thought to cause another 5,000 lung cancer deaths. Thus, if all Americans stopped smoking, 87 percent of lung cancer deaths could be prevented.

Lung cancer has the poorest five-year survival rate of all major cancers. In 1983, the five-year survival rate was only 13 percent, up slightly from 8 percent 20 years prior. In 1993, the survival rate is estimated to be around 14 percent.

But, I repeat: lung cancer can easily be prevented!

Now there must be a problem here. If it is so easily prevented, why is it number one and increasing in incidence in women?

Something isn't working. Smoking is the number-one cause of lung cancer. So not enough people have stopped smoking.

Cigarette manufacturers took advantage of the feminist movement to promote smoking in women. This was at the same time that men were starting to kick the habit. Due to the approximately 20-year lag time between smoking initiating the cancer process and the detection of lung cancer, women were soon on their way to achieving equality in the lung cancer race. However, men still hold the lead at around 70 per 100,000 for white males and near 95 per 100,000 for black males.

However, the rise isn't limited to women who smoke. More nonsmoking women were getting cancer in 1985 than all women combined 30 years earlier. The 1985 rate for lung cancer in women was 6.1 per 100,000 for nonsmokers and 26.4 for smokers. The rate for female smokers in 1988 increased further to 29.8 per 100,000. This compared to only 5.1 for all women in 1955.

The reason may be that women nonsmokers are now subjected to more secondhand smoke from their coworkers and friends, radon gas, and maybe air pollution.

At the same time, lung cancer death rates among white men appear to have peaked around 1988, and have been predicted to start a noticeable decline by the mid-1990s. The percentage of the U.S. population who smoke has dropped from 50 percent in 1965 to 25 percent in 1990.

As discussed in Chapter 7, antioxidant nutrients can protect against lung cancer. Please refer back to Table 7.1. Remember that the rate for lung cancer among moderate smokers who ate lots of beta-carotene and vitamin A is lower than among the nonsmokers who ate little beta-carotene and vitamin A.

Of course, I am not trying to tell you that you should continue to smoke and just take your vitamins. I am suggesting that you not smoke *and* take your vitamins. However, if you won't stop smoking, and have tried and tried and tried (heck, no one is perfect), then at least consider taking your vitamins.

I am not one to throw you to the dogs just because you don't do what is good for you. I want to keep you alive long enough so that you can try to quit smoking again sometime.

There is more to reducing the harm of cigarette smoke and radon than taking vitamin A and beta-carotene. Vitamin C, vitamin E, vitamin B12, folic acid, selenium and the sulfur-containing nutrients are all very important as well.

The following landmark studies show that these nutrients do protect against lung cancer. The study that I referred you to in Chapter 7 is the 1981 Western Electric study.[1] This was the 19-year study of 1,954 middle-aged men that surprised many researchers by finding that beta-carotene and vitamin A did protect against lung cancer, and as a result many other scientists started studying the effect.

Among 30-year smokers, lung cancer incidence decreased as the amount of beta-carotene in the diet increased: for those who consumed the least beta-carotene (100-3,700 IU), the lung cancer rate was 6.5 percent; for those who consumed 3,800-5,000 IU of beta-carotene, the lung cancer rate decreased to 4.5 percent; for those who consumed 5,100-6,600 IU, the cancer rate declined still further to 3.0 percent, and for those who ate *more than 6,700 IU of beta-carotene daily, the lung cancer rate dropped to 0.8 percent.*

This is a drop from 6.5 percent to 0.8 percent just with beta-carotene. If all of the antioxidant nutrients are taken in optimal amounts, the protection is much better due to synergism.

In 1990, Dr. Walter C. Willett of the Harvard School of Public Health reviewed this relationship in *Nutrition Reviews*.[2] His summary states in part, "In a dozen case-control and cohort studies, high intake of fruits and vegetables containing carotenoids has been associated with a reduced risk of lung cancer. . . . Available data thus strongly support the hypothesis that dietary carotenoids reduce the risk of lung cancer. . . ."

In 1986, Dr. Marilyn Menkes and her colleagues at Johns Hopkins did a case-control study of 99 lung cancer patients in Washington County, Maryland. They concluded: "These data support an association between low levels of serum vitamin E and the risk of any type of lung cancer and between low levels of serum beta-carotene and the risk of squamous-cell carcinoma of the lung."[3]

A Finnish study led by Dr. Paul Knekt of over 4,500 men over 20 years found that carotenoids and vitamins C and E have a protective effect.[4]

Radon

A word about radon, in case you are not familiar with this gas that accumulates in some homes. Radon is thought to be the third or fourth leading cause of cancer, with most estimates centering around 13,000 lung cancer deaths annually due to radon.

Radon is a radioactive gas that forms in some soils and travels upward into homes where it is trapped and accumulates in tightly sealed homes. The Environmental Protection Agency estimates that more than 20 million homes have dangerous levels of radon. Homes can be tested with kits available from local government agencies and even some hardware stores.

Although radon is a neutral gas, its radioactivity initiates free radicals. Radon arises from the radioactive decay of uranium, and many gravels and rocks, including granite and shale, contain traces of uranium. Radon gets its name from radium. Uranium 238 slowly decays radioactively to produce radium 226 and other by-products. The radon releases alpha particles (radiation), but lasts only a short time, having a half-life of 3.8 days. However, the decay products of radon, called radon progeny, are solids and can be inhaled and trapped in the lungs. Some of the radon progeny have very long radioactive lifetimes and can cause many, many free radicals to form in the lung tissues.

Prevention and Treatment of Lung Cancer

You can reduce your risk of cancer by being well-nourished and fortified with the antioxidant nutrients, as described earlier in this book. You should take a well-balanced multivitamin and mineral supplement, plus you may wish to take extra amounts of the following nutrients to obtain the following daily amounts:

beta-carotenes	10,000-30,000 IU
vitamin A	5,000-10,000 IU
vitamin E	200-800 IU

vitamin C	2,000–12,000 mg
selenium	100–200 mcg
N-acetylcysteine	250–1,000 mg
glutathione	as per label
cysteine or cystine	500–1,500 mg
folic acid	400–800 mcg
vitamin B12	50–100 mcg
pycnogenol	60–120 mg

The treatment strategy would be to immediately start a supplement program as above, followed by the best conventional treatment with shark cartilage as an adjunct.

REFERENCES

1. R. B. Shekelle et al., "Dietary vitamin A and risk of cancer in the Western Electric study," *Lancet* (1981) 2:1185-90.
2. Walter C. Willett, "Vitamin A and lung cancer," *Nutrition Reviews* (May, 1990) 48(5):201-211.
3. Marilyn S. Menkes et al., "Serum beta-carotene, vitamins A and E, selenium, and the risk of lung cancer," *New England Journal of Medicine* (Nov. 13, 1986) 315 (20): 1250-4.
4. Paul Knekt et al., "Dietary antioxidants and the risk of lung cancer," *American Journal of Epidemiology* (1991) 134 (5): 471-9.

CHAPTER 19

Breast Cancer

Not only is lung cancer incidence increasing in women, but so is breast cancer. Each year now, more than 180,000 women are being diagnosed as having breast cancer, and 46,000 women are dying due to breast cancer. Men can get breast cancer, too, but their numbers are not included in with the women's so that I can show the increase of breast cancer only for women. In 1940, we were told that the risk of a woman developing breast cancer was one in twenty. Now we are told that the risk is one in eight! Breast cancer incidence for women has climbed 26 percent in the 15 years between 1973 and 1988. In the 42 years between 1940 and 1982, the incidence of breast cancer in women climbed an average of 1.2 percent per year. And, there is no indication that the rate will stop increasing.

Just what does "risk" mean, and what does that have to do with any one person?

Risk

Talking about risk is a tricky thing. Sometimes public health officials use the statisticians' "risk" to scare the public into doing what the health officials think is best for them. As an example, if you hear that your risk of getting breast cancer is "one in eight," health officials believe that will encourage you to give yourself breast exams and have regular mammograms done.

I don't believe that these figures should be used to frighten the geeheepers out of you. Relax a little, take your vitamins, and get your checkups without fail. But, please don't go through life frightened to death. When they say that a women now has one chance in eight of getting breast cancer, that doesn't mean that if eight women are in a room, that one of them will certainly get breast cancer. Nor does it mean that in 8,000 women that 1,000 of them will get breast cancer.

Statistics can be deceiving and they are best used by statisticians. Let me make a few points about cancer risk. I saved this discussion for this chapter, because I am opposed to scaring people to motivate them, and I find nothing scarier than reading that one in eight women will get breast cancer.

The number of new cases of breast cancer reported each year between 1985 and 1990 averaged around 150,000. There are at least 128 million females in the U.S. If 180,000 of the 128,000,000 females get cancer each year, that is one in 711. If a women lives 80 years, then she runs the risk of 80 times one in 711, or a risk of one in 8.9 *over her lifetime if she reaches 80 years of age.*

Now statisticians use adjustment figures to consider the ages of all the females in the population, and the actual figures are slightly different, but the point is the same. Women have a risk of developing breast cancer in any given year that varies with their age, and a cumulative risk that accrues as they age. The one-in-eight figure combines all possible lifetimes of the women to predict that a girl born at this time, provided the incidence of cancer remains the same, will have a one-in-eight chance of developing breast cancer in her lifetime.

To me, more meaningful figures are that less than two percent (1.6) of all U.S. women who are 40 today will develop breast cancer by their 50th birthday. *That is one lady in 63.* Or, slightly more than two percent (2.4) of all U.S. women who are 50 years old today will develop breast cancer by their 60th birthday. That is still only one in 41. Or, between 60 and 70 years of age, 3.6 percent may develop breast cancer—one in 28. Or, between 70 and 80 years, 4.2 percent—one in 24. I can deal with these numbers better than one in eight.

However, I firmly believe that we can knock the incidence down to one-tenth of this, if all women eat adequate amounts of the antioxidant nutrients! And, we can cure many more of those who do develop breast cancer—male and female.

While we are talking about statistics and risk, let's consider another point. With some rare cancers, increasing the risk by 50 percent really doesn't mean much. But, with a common cancer, increasing the risk translates into many more people getting cancer. Let's say that the fictitious risk of a fictitious cancer, "xyz" cancer, is one in a zen dillion (a fictitious number). Since there are only several billion people on Earth, it seems unlikely that anyone will have "xyz" cancer. Doubling this risk will still not affect many people.

Now let's compare this to another fictitious risk of another fictitious cancer, "abc" cancer, which has a one in two risk. Already half of the world's population is at risk, and if the risk is increased by only 10 percent, millions of people will be affected.

My point is, that if you read that doing something you like increases your risk of cancer, evaluate just what that means to you. If eating your favorite food is associated with a 20-percent increase in risk of a certain cancer, look at the quantity of people involved. "Rate" is one thing, "quantity" is another.

If a million people who eat that food will have a total of two who develop cancer, compared to another million people who don't eat that food who will have only one person develop cancer, you can say that that food is associated with doubling the risk of cancer. But, if you really like that food, you may decide the risk is worth the chance that you will not be that one in a million who develops cancer. Thus, the risk (rate) is double, but in this case, the actual risk in terms of people is only one in a million.

In the case of breast cancer, the risk and numbers are both high, so we have to pay attention to all of the major risk factors.

Major Risk Factors

There have been many studies of breast cancer risk factors, and unfortunately, some of them contradict others. When this is the case, it either means that the studies were inadequately designed or that the factor being evaluated is actually a secondary factor or co-risk factor of another unrecognized factor. I'll try to sort some of these out.

Let's start with the obvious. Of course, like just about everything else, age and family history are risk factors, but there is not too much we can do to change either. Even here, there is some confusion because the term "family history of cancer" is often misinterpreted. Dr. Walter Willett of Harvard and his research group have summarized these risk factors very nicely:

"A family history of breast cancer, particularly when the diagnosis was made in the mother, sister or daughter at a young age, can be an important risk factor for breast cancer. As compared with the risk among women not having a mother, sister or daughter (first-degree relative) with breast cancer, overall the relative risk is on the order of 1.5 to 2 for women who have one first-degree relative with breast cancer and may be as high as 4 to 6 for those with two affected first-degree relatives. (Note: Aunts are not first-degree relatives.)

"The risks are heightened if the cancer was bilateral. For a woman with a sister who had bilateral cancer before the age of 50, the lifetime cumulative risk of breast cancer appears to be greater than 50 percent, and is even higher if the sister was affected before the age of 40.

"The excess relative risk declines with the age of the relative at the time of diagnoses. For a woman whose mother had unilateral breast cancer after the age of 60, the excess relative risk is only about 40 percent greater than that associated with having no first-degree relatives with breast cancer."[1]

Other risk factors that we don't have much control over include early menarche (first menstruation), age at the birth of the first child, and late menopause. Girls who have menarche before 12 years of age have about a 20 percent increase in risk compared to those who have menarche at 14 years or older.

Women who have their first child after the age of 30 or who have no children have twice the risk of breast cancer as those who have their first child before the age of 20. As the number of women who postpone families until later in life increases, these figures may change as well. They could turn out to be statistical aberrations due to the comparatively limited numbers involved. By the way, the number of births seems to have no effect on breast cancer risk.

Women who have natural menopause after the age of 55 have twice the risk of breast cancer as those who begin menopause before 45 years of age.

Oral Contraceptives, Estrogen Replacement Therapy and Risk

A controversial item is whether or not the use of estrogen in birth control pills or postmenopausal therapy increases the risk of breast cancer. According to Dr. Willett's group in 1992, the use of oral contraceptives appears to increase the risk of breast cancer by about 50 percent, but the excess risk drops rapidly after the drug is discontinued.[1] They note that "in several case-control studies among women younger than 45 years of age, the use of oral contraceptives for more than a few years was associated with increases in risk irrespective of when they were used."[1]

Another review of twelve previous studies concluded that the use of oral contraceptives for four years or less did not increase the risk of breast cancer.[2]

Still many other studies showed either no link or a link only to early-onset breast cancer which is relatively rare. In fact, the majority of the studies show no link between "the pill" and breast cancer.[2] Other scientists point out the studies used to link oral contraceptives to breast cancer involved women who entered the study program many years ago when the amount of estrogen used in birth control pills was much higher, and that the newer pills are much safer. Some earlier studies even claim that oral contraceptives are protective against breast cancer.

So this issue may still be unresolved in spite of the existing copious amounts of existing data. Only time will tell. Keep in mind that breast cancer incidence is rising quickly and no one seems to have an explanation for it.

Postmenopausal therapy with estrogen also seems to increase the risk of cancer by about 40 percent, according to Dr. Willett's group. Combining progesterone with the estrogen does seem to decrease the risk of endometrial cancer, but does not appear to decrease the risk of breast cancer and may even add to the risk.[1,3,4]

It is obvious that female hormones have an effect on at least one type of breast cancer, and this will be discussed further later in this chapter.

Cystic Mastitis, Other Benign Breast Diseases and Risk

Now we come to another confusing issue—benign breast disease. Benign breast disease is a term that includes many different diseases. The lay person can be very confused by the terms benign breast disease, cystic mastitis, fibrocystic breast disease, mammary dysplasia, and lobular cancer *in situ*. (*In situ* literally means "in place or position." Here it describes a non-invasive tumor that "stays in place.") Other mystifying terms include ductal carcinoma *in situ* and proliferate breast disease. If you have a lump of any kind in your breast, have it checked by a physician. Most likely it is due to one of the above benign diseases, but you must be sure—do it as soon as possible!

I believe that benign lumps may hide malignant lumps that then go undetected in a woman's self-examination, or she may ignore a malignant lump because in the past, all that was found were benign lumps. These factors may increase the severity of a malignancy by allowing it to go undetected for a longer time.

If you do have a benign breast disease, even if the lumps are painful, it doesn't mean that you are at a higher risk for breast cancer, as some people think. A study by Drs. William Dupont and David Page found that 70 percent of the women with benign breast disease are not at increased risk for breast cancer.[5] The remaining 30 percent who either have a family history of breast cancer or who also have unusual lesions (abnormal tissues) may be at increased risk. Women who have proliferate epithelial changes have twice the risk of breast cancer, and women who have atypical hyperplasia have four times the risk. (Of women who have biopsies taken, only 4 to 10 percent are found to have atypical hyperplasia.) All of the others have no increased risk.

I hope that this is reassuring, because one of my pet peeves are those surgeons who advocate the surgical removal of breasts to prevent the occurrence of cancer. I still remember reading in 1980 where a surgeon was claiming he saved the life of a symptom-free young girl by removing both of her breasts. This may be an option on very rare occasions, but with our early detection methods and close monitoring, even most high-risk women need not resort to such drastic measures as a prophylactic. It seems more prudent to me to depend on antioxidant nutrients and the other dietary factors discussed in this chapter for prophylaxis.

Nipple Discharge

Many people think that the first sign of breast cancer is a lump. Just as often, early warning signs can include a steady ache in the breast, or a lump under the armpit (which is actually breast tissue that extends into that area), or a discharge from the nipple that persists for more than a couple of weeks. Another warning sign is a dimpling of the skin that lasts for more than a couple of days. Of course, a postmenopausal woman who has a new ache in a breast should see her physician.

However, nipple discharge that is expressed during examination of a breast is not unusual, and usually not a sign of trouble. Many women are properly trained to squeeze their nipples during self-examination to test for discharge. In many women, there will be a discharge, and the more they squeeze to test, the more discharge is produced. About 80 percent of all women will produce a discharge if they are suctioned with a special device used by physicians.

In order for nipple discharge to be a concern, it must be unrelated to pregnancy or breast-feeding; in addition, it must come from the ducts themselves without mechanical stimulation, and regularly for at least several weeks.[6]

Body Shape and Risk

There are studies and there are studies. Some studies suggest that height may be a risk factor. I discount this as merely reflecting that breast cancer occurs more often in Westernized societies, which also have taller ladies. I don't believe that this is a cause-and-effect situation.

However, genetics do play a role in how each individual stores body fat. As an example, ladies can be divided into two classes when they put on those extra pounds. Some store a more than average percentage of their fat below their waist in their derrieres and thighs, while the others tend to accumulate their extra fat around their waistline and upper body (central adiposity). The former type are often referred to as being pear-shaped and the latter as being apple-shaped. Pear-shaped ladies are more prone to adult-onset diabetes and apple-shaped ladies are more prone to developing heart disease.

Now there is an indication that apple-shaped ladies are also at a slightly greater risk of developing breast cancer. Women with waist-to-hip ratios above a certain level have more breast cancer than those who have lower levels.

The correct way to measure the waist-to-hip ratio for assessing this risk factor is to measure the hips at their widest circumference and the waist at the navel. Be sure to keep the measuring tape parallel to the floor and free of twists. The ratio is obtained by dividing the size of your waist by your hip size (W/H).

If your waist-to-hip ratio is above 0.81, your risk of breast cancer may be *seven times greater* than if the ratio is less than 0.73.[7] Sorry to bring it up, but, the smaller your waist, the lower your risk of breast cancer. And a factor that increases the risk seven times is a very, very significant factor!

This also makes sense biochemically. There are connections related to free radicals in stored body fat and also estrogen levels. So part of this risk may be genetic (where the fat is deposited) and part of the risk may be a factor that you can control (the amount of fat stored).

Risk Factors You Can Control

In spite of the study that showed that obesity seemed to protect younger women against breast cancer, the *amount of fat stored around the waist seems to be a large risk factor*. This is partly because fat increases the number of cancer-causing free radicals and the amount of estrogen. Why waist-stored fat is worse than hip-stored fat is not known, but it may have something to do with the fact that upper-body fat also includes the breasts themselves, and the more fat stored in the breast, the more likely that that breast tissue will be affected by the fat. Also there is evidence that central adiposity results in more estrogen being freely available and not bound in globin.

So, with this very significant risk factor there are three things that you can do to protect yourself. First, keep the waistline fat to a reasonable minimum. Second, take antioxidant nutrients to destroy the excess free radicals produced from this extra fat. Third, keep your total estrogen level from exceeding normal limits.

You can accomplish these goals by practicing moderation. There is no need to be fashion-model thin. Being thin at the expense of eating good foods and a balanced diet is counter-productive. A diet of diet sodas and small salads will not nourish you sufficiently to protect you from cancer. Good wholesome food, low in fat, high in fiber, exercise and daily supplements will be your best strategy to keep your waist-to-hip ratio below 0.73 *and you in your best health*!

As far as your total estrogens go, if your waist-to-hip ratio exceeds 0.81, then be wary of taking extra estrogen such as in oral contraceptives or postmenopausal therapy pills. Have your blood estrogen level monitored by your physician. If your waistline-to-hip ratio is less than 0.73, then just take your vitamins and don't worry.

Now let's go back and consider: what if your waist-to-hip ratio isn't quite perfect? Or, if it is, you may be struggling to keep it perfect. One important factor is the amount of fat in your diet, and of course, this is also reflected in the number of calories in your diet.

Dietary Fat and Risk

If waist-to-hip ratio can influence breast cancer risk by sevenfold, then it is not surprising that dietary fat or total calories may be involved. Let's look at what we know in 1993.

Here again we have many studies with conflicting confusions. We can throw out the studies comparing the fat intake of various cultures to their incidence of breast cancer. There are just too many confounding variables not considered by these studies.

Studies of members of the same culture, as these members migrate to a new culture and have their incidence of breast cancer dramatically change, have more bearing on the factors being studied and fewer confounding factors. These studies generally support the premise that increasing amounts of dietary fat in the diet are associated with an increasing incidence of breast cancer.

Still there are many confounding factors in these "migration" studies because the migration is usually to more affluent countries. The factors of affluence—labor-saving devices, less physical work, more dietary calories, less dietary fiber, more leisure time, pollution, etc.—all lead to a greater accumulation of body fat, and hence, a poorer waist-to-hip ratio.

Then there are the longitudinal cohort studies that follow the same women over many years and then compare the diets of the women who get breast cancer to similar women who don't get breast cancer. One such large ongoing study is headed by Harvard researcher Dr. Walter Willett. Dr. Willett's group has been studying 89,000 nurses since 1980.

In 1987, they published their first report and concluded that dietary fat was not related to the incidence of breast cancer.[8] In 1992, they published a follow-up study that again concluded after investigating the diets of 1,439 breast cancer patients and comparing their diets to healthy nurses matched in age and other factors, that there was no link between dietary fat and breast cancer.[9]

Dr. Willett's group summarized their data as "these data provide evidence against both an adverse influence of fat intake and a protective effect of fiber consumption by middle-aged women on breast cancer incidence. . . . Our findings suggest that, among middle-aged women, a moderate decrease in fat intake, as advised by numerous official groups, will not substantially reduce breast cancer incidence."[9]

This type of study can be more meaningful to U.S. women, because it evaluates the diets of women who have similar lifestyles and food habits. Unfortunately, the studies also have their limitations, as they are based on questionnaires usually given either at the beginning of the studies or at the end, and there is no way to detect changes in the diet that may occur during the many years of the studies. Also, some scientists feel that these studies consider only women having typical American diets; thus, even the best diets are poor because they contain too much fat.

As an example, in the nurses study, dietary fat ranged from 32 to 44 percent of the total diet calories. Many researchers believe that a protective effect from a lower fat diet will not begin to appear until the fat content of the diet dips below 25 percent of total calories.

Another cohort study of 5,485 women, of whom 99 developed breast cancer, actually suggested that higher fat diets had a protective effect against breast cancer.[10] However, this protective effect was not statistically significant.

A third study, an epidemiological study, also found no link between dietary fat and breast cancer. Researchers at Loma Linda University studied 20,000 Seventh Day Adventist women for six years. During that time, 215 cases of breast cancer were diagnosed, with the average age being 66 years. Although most of the other risk factors mentioned earlier applied, there was no association with dietary fat or total dietary calories.

The women who were vegetarians from early childhood had no less risk than those women who became vegetarians as adults.[11]

A fourth study, a case-control study of 183 sets of Japanese women and 161 sets of Caucasian women, found no statistically significant differences between those with breast cancer and their matched controls in terms of dietary fat, saturated fat, animal protein, cholesterol, and two individual fatty acids. The researchers concluded that "if there is an association of dietary fat with breast cancer, it is not a strong one."[12]

Thus, epidemiological studies and cohort studies are limited, and there appear to be conflicting opinions. However, until proper clinical trials are conducted (and there are so many problems in getting two large groups of women to maintain the same diets for 20 years that these studies may never be made), we have to rely more heavily on laboratory animal studies than we would normally like to do. After all, there are important differences.

In the case of most laboratory animal studies, dietary fat is implicated with increased risk of breast cancer. But, even here, there is debate as to whether or not the increased risk is due to fat *per se,* or to total calories. The preponderance of the evidence seems to support the premise that both dietary fat *per se,* total calories and body fat are all equal culprits. By dietary fat, I mean all types of fat—saturated and polyunsaturated fats alike.

In fact, my studies in the early 1970s indicated that polyunsaturated fats are great promoters of cancer because they contribute to free-radical production.[13] As mentioned earlier, dietary fats and increased body fat also increase estrogen production and estrogen receptors in cells. In addition, fats increase carcinogenic estrogen metabolites.[14] Fats also affect prostaglandin production, which could possibly play a role in cancer. Another very important consideration is that fat depresses the immune system. There is evidence that dietary fat and body fat can affect the growth and spread of cancer. We will discuss this later under therapy.

So, to summarize the dietary fat debate, the bulk of the good evidence at this writing seems to link both dietary fat and total calories to breast cancer incidence. However, the strength of this evidence is statistically weak, there are conflicting studies, and future studies could challenge this association. Science and truth aren't decided by the number of studies, but by the quality of the studies. At this point, there isn't enough quality evidence to unequivocally determine this issue for breast cancer.

But, we have to go on the best evidence that we have, and if we err, we must err on the conservative side—the side that will do least harm if later proven wrong. My advice is that at this time you can choose to go on a low-fat (15-25 percent) diet, or to just keep in mind the waist-to-hip ratio discussed earlier, go easy on the fats and total calories, and most important of all, take adequate amounts of the antioxidant nutrients.

Exercise

Of course, if body fat is a risk factor, lack of activity or exercise is also a risk factor as it allows your metabolism to slow and makes it easier to put on fat. The more lean muscle tissue you have in your body, the more little calorie-burning factories, called mitochondria, you have to use up calories, even when you are not using your muscles. Epidemiological studies confirm this relationship. The more you exercise, the lower your risk of breast cancer.

Fiber and Risk

People often associate dietary fiber with reducing the rate of colon cancer, but few are aware of its role in breast cancer. I have mentioned fiber as being beneficial in low-fat, high-fiber diets, but high-fiber diets offer additional protection regardless of whether the fat content is high or low.

Drs. Leonard Cohen and Ernst L. Wynder of the American Health Foundation have found that when bran, a high-fiber food, is added to a high-fat diet (40 percent fat, 5 percent fiber) given to laboratory rats who are also injected with a chemical carcinogen, the rate of induced breast cancer drops form 90 percent to 67 percent. The amount of bran added to the 40-percent fat diet (typical of the standard U.S. diet) doubled the existing 5 percent fiber to ten percent.

They also fed half of the rats a low-fat diet (10 percent fat, 5 percent fiber). When half of the laboratory rats on the low-fat diet had their fiber content doubled to ten percent, their rates of induced breast cancer dropped from 63 percent to 47 percent.

Low-fat, high-fiber diet proponents recommend a diet having 10 *percent* of total calories as fat and including 45 *grams* of fiber. However, most experts realize that most Americans simply will not eat this type of diet, so realizing the facts of the real world, they strive for a diet that is no more than 25 percent fat and having 25 grams or more of dietary fiber. This is often called the 25/25 diet. I will discuss dietary fiber and fiber-rich foods more fully in the next chapter, on colon cancer.

Alcohol and Risk

It would be nice to be able to tell you that at least the link between alcohol consumption and breast cancer is clear-cut. It is to me, but unfortunately, there are a few conflicting studies that can't be ignored. Based on my experience with laboratory animal studies, alcohol is a promoter (although not an initiator) of breast cancer, and the degree of cancer promotion is directly related to the amount of alcohol in the diet.

Indeed, the vast majority of the reliable studies, sixteen of twenty, show that alcohol consumption is linked to risk of breast cancer. The only issue in the reports showing a direct linkage is whether or not there is a threshold alcohol intake such that being below that threshold results in no additional risk and being above that level does mean an increased risk. The reports are fairly evenly divided in number, but I feel that the better quality studies indicate that, as with the animal studies, the risk is in direct proportion to the amount of alcohol consumed.

The following are representative of those studies showing a statistically significant link between alcohol consumption and breast cancer. If these studies are correct, then heavy drinking is a very serious risk factor for breast cancer. (In these studies, a "drink" is usually defined as 12 ounces of beer, a glass of wine, or a drink having 1 ounce of alcohol.) Let's start with the nurses survey, since these 89,000-plus nurses have provided so much information for us.

Dr. Walter Willett and his Harvard research group found no increased risk of breast cancer for women who drank less than three drinks per day (5 grams of alcohol).[15] For women drinking between three and nine drinks daily (5 to 14 grams of alcohol), there was a 30 percent increase in risk. With the breast cancer incidence so high, that is a serious rise with meaning for many, many women. For women drinking ten or more drinks per day (15 grams or more), there was a 60 percent jump in breast cancer risk. Of course, the data were adjusted to account for confounding factors such as smoking, body weight, and all known risk factors.

The "NHANES" follow-up study was published in the same journal issue and is in good agreement. The data obtained in the National Health and Nutrition Examination Survey from 7,188 women aged 25 to 74 years were followed up after ten years.[16] During that time 121 women developed breast cancer.

Using non-drinkers as a baseline, the study reported that there was a 50-percent increase in breast cancer risk for women drinking any amount of alcohol at all. When the data are broken down into three levels of alcohol consumption, the increases in risk are as follows; any -1.3 grams of alcohol daily increased risk by 40 percent, 1.3-4.9 grams of alcohol daily increased risk by 50 percent, and more than five grams of alcohol daily (about three drinks) increased risk by 60 percent.

The researchers reported that the association between drinking and breast cancer was stronger among younger, leaner, premenopausal women. They concluded that, *"moderate alcohol consumption is associated with an elevation in the risk of breast cancer of 50 to 100 percent."*

Remember that an increase in risk of 100 percent means that the risk is doubled. If you are already uncomfortable with the statistic that one in eight women will develop breast cancer, then doubling your risk means that the risk is now one in four! I would think that if you are already at higher risk than normal because of things you can't control, then you might consider not drinking alcohol except maybe on very rare occasions. In other words, high-risk women should not drink or should drink only moderately, unless some startling new information surfaces stating otherwise.

A third study agreeing closely with the "NHANES" study drew from a data bank of 68,674 women.[17] By 1984, 303 of the healthy "study" women had developed breast cancer. After controlling for the confounding factors of age, race, body mass, smoking and other known risk factors, drinkers were found to have a 50-percent increase in breast cancer risk. Those who drank one to two drinks daily had a 50-percent increase in risk, as did those who drank three to five drinks per day. However, *those who drank six or more drinks daily had three and a third times the risk of breast cancer!*

A fourth study, a case-control study of 1,524 breast cancer patients and 1,892 matched controls also found that breast cancer risk increased as daily consumption of alcohol increased.[18] After adjusting for known risk factors, there was a strong association between moderate alcohol consumption in early life and subsequent breast cancer. One to two drinks per day increased risk by 30 percent, while *consuming more than two drinks per day increased risk by 70 percent.*

As I said, there are at least 20 good studies at this writing, and they are not all as conclusive for the moderate drinking findings. A "meta" study—a study that combines data from several studies—of six case-control studies, concludes that there is no significant increase in risk for moderate drinkers (less than three alcoholic drinks per day). The risk for those drinking more than three drinks daily increases by 70 percent.[19] I am not a fan of "meta" analyses, since the conditions in the various studies being grouped together can sometimes be so different as to blur the data.

As for the studies absolving alcohol, the evidence is less convincing. In 1990, a Canadian group repeated their 1982 study and found the same results—no statistically significant linkage—using a larger number of women in their newer study.[20] However, an increase in risk of breast cancer of 70 percent was observed for women who drank at least one beer daily, although the data were not statistically significant. This study also found that women who drank at least one glass of wine daily had a 30 percent reduction in breast cancer incidence. (Could this be due to the protective effect of bioflavonoids in wine?) This study could suffer from selection bias and inadequate control for confounding factors, however.

Similarly, in 1989, a group at the U.S. Centers for Disease Control (CDC) taking part in the "Cancer and Steroid Hormone Study" also tested their 1983 finding of no linkage between alcohol consumption and breast cancer incidence. Their larger study included an additional 2,272 breast cancer cases and 1,978 controls. Based on questionnaires, the researchers reported that women who drank any alcohol at all had no difference in risk of breast cancer than nondrinkers.[21]

Smoking and Risk

Smoking is well accepted as a cause or contributing factor to several cancers, but it is *usually* absolved as a significant risk factor for breast cancer. Some researchers even feel that smoking might reduce estrogen levels and that could have some protective effect.[22] However, there are two research reports that deserve greater attention and additional studies.

Both studies use sophisticated data analyses. One study indicates a significant risk of breast cancer for smokers, and the other study strongly suggests that smokers have greater cancer spread and greater recurrence.

Researchers at the University of British Columbia used data collected from 31,000 women in the Canadian National Breast Screening Study.[23] Dr. Martin Schechter and his research team found a 260 percent *increase* in breast cancer incidence for premenopausal women who currently smoked at the time of cancer detection. That's 3.6 times the normal risk! The increased risk among postmenopausal women was 30 percent, except among postmenopausal women having no children, who had an increased risk of 190 percent (2.9 times normal). This may suggest an interaction with hormones that produces carcinogenic metabolites.

The researchers found that there was a strong trend towards increasing risk of breast cancer with the increasing number of cigarettes smoked daily. The study considered many confounding factors including frequency of breast examination, previous mammograms, level of education, family history, age at birth of first child, benign breast disease, and history of breast lumps, pain or discharge.

Add this study to that of Dr. Jean Hager and her colleagues at the AMC Cancer Research Center in Denver. They have found that nonsmokers have a 10 percent rate of metastasis two years after mastectomy, while smokers have a 30 percent rate.[24] They also found that four years after mastectomy, smokers had a 40 percent incidence of metastasis, whereas nonsmokers had only an 18 percent incidence.

Dr. Hager concludes, "our data indicate smoking is a big risk in breast cancer." Let me remind you that smoking is also a big risk in many cancers.

Antioxidant Nutrients

As I mentioned in Chapter 10 on selenium, I believe that the incidence of breast cancer could be reduced to only 10 percent of its present level if all women would take optimal amounts of selenium and other antioxidant nutrients. One case-control study examined the protective effect of dietary selenium and beta-carotene, along with a low-fat, high-fiber diet, and found that this diet reduced the incidence of breast cancer to 40 percent of normal.[25] However, even this good diet was not optimized, as it included no supplements to bring the protective antioxidant nutrients up to their optimal levels.

I will briefly review the major antioxidant nutrients that are protective against cancer. They were discussed more fully in their separate chapters in the first section of this book. Remember, they work best in combination.

SELENIUM

Dr. Gerhard Schrauzer of the University of California at San Diego conducted a joint study with colleagues at the National Cancer Center Hospital in Tokyo.[26] Blood samples were drawn from healthy women in both the United States and Japan and also from women having either breast cancer, recurrent breast cancer or benign breast disease. The blood samples were coded and then sent to a laboratory for selenium analyses.

As it turned out, the healthy Japanese women had the highest levels of selenium in their blood (0.286 mcg/ml), while Japanese women with benign breast disease had 0.200 mcg/ml and breast cancer patients had 0.195 mcg/ml. Healthy American women had 0.191 micrograms of selenium per milliliter of blood, while American women having benign breast disease had 0.142 mcg/ml and breast cancer patients had 0.167 mcg/ml.

However, the lowest of all blood selenium levels were from the recurrent breast cancer patients. The difference in the absolute values between the women in each country can be attributed to differences in diet, but the important thing is that women with lower than normal levels of selenium in their blood compared to the normal level for their country had a greater risk of breast cancer.

This difference in blood selenium levels can be a clue as to whether or not a patient has breast cancer or not within a country. In 1990, Drs. Helena Krsnjavi and Dubravka Beker of the Yugoslavian Institute of Medical Research in Zagreb measured the level of selenium in the blood of breast cancer patients, benign breast disease patients and healthy women. They found the level in blood of breast cancer patients was markedly lower (41-58 mcg/l) than that of the healthy women (73-89 mcg/l) and those with benign breast disease (67-76 mcg/l.)[27]

As I mention in Chapter 10, there are many, many studies showing that selenium is protective against breast cancer. There are also occasional epidemiological studies showing no relationship of dietary selenium to breast cancer, but these studies are seriously flawed in that they depend on book values for food selenium content, and foods vary tremendously in selenium content depending on the region in which they are grown.

VITAMIN E

Vitamin E is selenium's partner, and the combined effect of vitamin E and selenium in protecting against breast cancer is discussed in Chapters 9 and 10.

Vitamin C

Chapter 8 discusses the role of vitamin C in preventing various types of cancers. Pertaining to breast cancer, the evidence typically shows what Dr. Geoffrey Howe of the National Cancer Institute of Canada found in a meta-analysis of twelve studies on diet and breast cancer.[28] He suggests that consuming at least 380 milligrams of vitamin C daily could reduce breast cancer incidence by 16 percent. Now this is a case of more *is* better. See the recommendations near the end of this chapter.

Vitamin D and Calcium

One of the most interesting discoveries is that breast cancer and colon cancer incidences are lower in the sunbelts and in rural areas. This fortuitous discovery by Dr. Cedrick Garland is described in Chapter 14, but I will cite another confirming study here.

Researchers at the University of Western Ontario and Memorial Sloan-Kettering Cancer Center in New York studied the roles of vitamin D and calcium in chemical carcinogen-induced breast cancer in laboratory rats.[29] They studied vitamin D and calcium separately and together.

The researchers found that vitamin D and calcium had interactive effects on breast cancer prevention. High intakes of vitamin D inhibited the growth of tumors when calcium and phosphorus intakes were low. They also found that a low intake of vitamin D and/or high intake of phosphorus reduces calcium bioavailability and increases the risk for breast cancer.

Prevention of Breast Cancer

The prevention of breast cancer depends, more than anything else, on being well-nourished with antioxidant nutrients. One of the roles of the antioxidant nutrients is to prevent the damage done by both dietary fat and body fat. Of course, lowering the fat content of the diet and total calories in the diet is helpful, too, as long as optimal nourishment is obtained. In other words, diet colas, lettuce and toast as your total diet is low-calorie and low-fat, but by themselves, these foods do not supply adequate nourishment to protect against cancer, and the net result would be an increase in risk of all cancers.

As mentioned in the discussion on dietary fat, the 25/25 diet (no more than 25 *percent* of total calories as fat, and more than 25 *grams* of fiber) is a good target because it is practical. However, even the 25/25 diet needs antioxidant supplementation. You may wish to consider the following supplements.

NUTRIENT	AMOUNT
selenium	200 mcg
vitamin C	1,250-11,000 mg
vitamin E	400-800 IU
vitamin D	400 IU
calcium	400-1,000 mg
beta-carotene	10,000-15,000 IU
vitamin A	5,000-7,500 IU
iodine	150 mcg
folic acid	800 mcg
niacin or niacinamide	25-100 mg
magnesium	250-500 mg

The following are optional, but worth considering:

pycnogenol	30-60 mg
garlic	1-3 capsules
evening primrose oil	2 capsules
fish oil	1 capsule
canthaxanthin	1 capsule

Breast Cancer Treatment

Conventional therapy is your first choice of treatment, followed by shark cartilage therapy after about four to six weeks. You should nourish your immune system as described earlier and fight metastasis with the same preventive strategy mentioned above. There is some preliminary suggestion that rubbing a vitamin D cream on the skin over nodules of advanced or cutaneous metastatic breast cancer is promising. Please re-read Chapter 16 on shark cartilage and check to see what new information is available since this writing.

If surgery is suggested, be sure to ask the surgeon about the importance of timing the surgery to just before and during ovulation. Remember that better results are obtained after surgery if you stay on a low-fat diet, don't smoke, and take your supplements.

REFERENCES

1. Jay R. Harris et al., "Breast cancer: part one," *New England Journal of Medicine* (Aug. 13, 1992) 327(7):473-80.
2. Richard W. Sattin et al., "Oral contraceptive use and the risk of breast cancer," *New Engl. J. Med.* (Aug. 14, 1986) 315(7):405-11.
3. L. Bergkvist et al., "The risk of breast cancer after estrogen and estrogen-progestin replacement," *New Engl. J. Med.* (1989) 321:293-7.
4. G. A. Colditz et al., "Prospective study of estrogen-replacement therapy and the risk of breast cancer in postmenopausal women," *Journal of the American Medical Association* (1990) 264:2648-53.
5. D. William Dupont and David L. Page, *New Engl. J. Med.* (Jan. 17, 1985) 312:146-51.
6. William L. Donegan, Frederick L. Greene, and Susan M. Love, "Nipple discharge: is it cancer?" *Patient Care* (Jan. 30, 1990) 24:79.
7. P. F. Bruning et al., "Body measurements, estrogen availability and the risk of human breast cancer: a case-control study," *International Journal of Cancer* (Apr. 22, 1992) 51(1):14-9.
   Also see: *Annals of Internal Medicine* (1990) 112:182-6.
8. Walter C. Willett, et al., "Dietary fat and the risk of breast cancer," *New Engl. J. Med.* (1987) 316(1):22-8.

9. Walter C. Willett et al., "Dietary fat and fiber in relation to risk of breast cancer," *JAMA* (Oct. 21, 1992) 268(15):2037-44.

10. D. Yvonne Jones et al., "Dietary fat and breast cancer in the National Health and Nutritional Examination Survey Epidemiologic Follow-up Study," *Journal of the National Cancer Institute* (1987) 79:465-71.

11. P. Mills et al., "Dietary habits and breast cancer incidence among Seventh-Day Adventists," *Cancer* (1989) 64:582-90.

12. T. Hirohata et al., "An epidemiologic study on the association between diet and breast cancer," *Journal of the National Cancer Institute* (April 1987) 78(4):595-600.

13. Richard A. Passwater, "Cancer: new directions," *American Laboratory* (1973) 5(6):10-22.

14. C. Longcope et al., "The effect of a low-fat diet on estrogen metabolism," *Journal of Clinical Endocrinology* (1987) 64:1246-50.

15. Walter C. Willett et al., "Moderate alcohol consumption and the risk of breast cancer," *New Engl. J. Med.* (May 7, 1987) 316(19):1174-80.

16. A. Schatzkin et al., "Alcohol consumption and breast cancer in the Epidemiologic Follow-Up Study of the First National Health and Nutrition Examination Survey," *New Engl. J. Med.* (May 7, 1987) 316(19):1169-73.

17. R. A. Hiatt, A. L. Klatsky, and M. A. Armstrong, "Alcohol consumption and the risk of breast cancer in a prepaid health plan," *Cancer Research* (April 15, 1988) 48(8):2284-2287.

18. E.B. Harvey et al., "Alcohol consumption and breast cancer," *Journal of the National Cancer Institute* (April 1987) 78(4):657-61.

19. Geoffrey Howe et al., "The association between alcohol and breast cancer risk: evidence from the combined analysis of six dietary case-control studies," *International Journal of Cancer* (March 12, 1991) 47(5):707-10.

20. Lynn Rosenberg et al., "A case-control study of alcoholic beverage consumption and breast cancer," *American Journal of Epidemiology* (Jan. 1990) 131(1):6-14.

21. Susan Y. Chu et al., "Alcohol consumption and the risk of breast cancer," *American Journal of Epidemiology* (Nov. 1989) 130(5):867-77.

22. L. Berta et al., "Smoking effects on the hormonal balance of fertile women," *Hormone Research* (1992) 37:45-8.

23. Martin T. Schechter et al., "The relationship of cigarette smoking and breast cancer in the Canadian National Breast Screening Study," *Amer. J. Epidemiol.* (April, 1985) 121(4):479-87.

24. Jean C. Hager et al., "Cancer recurrence after mastectomy," reported in *Medical World News* (April 22, 1985) p. 13-14.
25. Pieter Van't Veer et al., "Combination of dietary factors in relation to breast cancer occurrence," *International Journal of Cancer* (March 12, 1991) 47(5):649-53.
26. Gerhard N. Schrauzer et al., "Selenium in the blood of japanese and american women with and without breast cancer and fibrocystic disease." *Japanese Journal of Cancer Research* (May, 1985) 76(5):374-7.
27. Helena Krsnjavi and Dubravka Beker, "Selenium in serum as a possible parameter for assessment of breast disease," *Breast Cancer Research and Treatment* (1990) 16(10):57-61.
28. Geoffrey R. Howe et al., "Dietary factors in risk of breast cancer: combined analysis of 12 case-control studies," *Journal of the National Cancer Institute* (1990) 82:561-69.
29. K. Carroll et al., "Calcium and carcinogenesis of the mammary gland," *American Journal of Clinical Nutrition* (1991) 54:2068-2088.

CHAPTER 20

Colon Cancer

The mystery of colon cancer has been solved. There were some surprises where at first seemingly unrelated clues were suddenly found to be interrelated and co-dependent. Before we look at the answer, let's look at the problem.

Worldwide, nearly half a million new cases of colon cancer occur annually. In 1987, approximately 60,000 Americans died from cancers of the colon (large intestine or bowel), rectum and anus, while about 145,000 new cases were reported. At that time, the National Cancer Institute estimated that 6 percent of the nearly 250 million U.S. citizens alive at that time would develop colon cancer and that six million of those would die of colon cancer.

Diet plays a major role in colon cancer, especially among those who are genetically susceptible. I discussed the role of genetics and how the colon cancer gene can be activated in Chapter 5, What Causes Cancer? We hear a lot about dietary fats and fiber, but they are the secondary factors. We now know what the primary factors are and which dietary factors affect them, and now we can zero-in more precisely with our preventive strategy.

It is not surprising that diet is a major contributing factor in colon cancer. After all, "colon" is just another word for "large intestine," and our food is digested in our intestines. If bad diet increases the risk, then good diet and/or supplements decreases the risk.

The colon is normally about 5 to 7 feet long. It starts at the

153

end of the small intestine and winds up the right side of the abdominal cavity (this part of the colon is called the ascending colon); crosses over the top of the abdominal cavity to the left side (this part is called the transverse colon); continues down the left side (the descending colon); and finally takes an S-shaped loop (sigmoid colon) to the rectum, which is normally about a foot long, and terminates at the anus.

About 50 percent of colorectal cancers are in the rectum, 20 percent in the sigmoid colon, 15 percent in the ascending colon, 6 to 8 percent in the transverse colon, 6 to 7 percent in the descending colon and 1 percent in the anus. The types of cancers found in the colon are adenocarcinoma, carcinoma, and squamous-cell (epidermoid) carcinoma.

This information on the cancer sites and types suggests that prolonged contact with certain chemicals is involved in the cancer process. The question then becomes, "Do the chemicals responsible for colon cancer come from the diet or are they produced in the body, or both?"

Many epidemiological studies have linked high-fat, low-fiber diets with colon cancer. In the preceding chapter I mentioned that vitamin D and calcium were protective against both breast cancer and colon cancer. There are studies that show that the antioxidant nutrients are protective against colon cancer as well. How then is diet responsible, if colon cancer is caused by the increased absorption of cancer-causing chemicals through the colon walls?

Although colon cancer can be produced in laboratory animals by the absorption of a number of chemicals that are not a part of our diets, most scientists believe that this is not the way colon cancer is caused in humans. The vast majority of human colon cancers are due primarily to chemicals that are byproducts of the *decomposition of* bacteria and excess dietary fat and bile in the colon.

A low-fiber diet contributes to colon cancer by slowing down the system so that these decomposition products linger in the colon for extended periods. This increases the length of time that these decomposed products are in contact with the colon and increases the amount that is absorbed into colon cells.

We learned in Chapter 14 that calcium protects the colon by

normalizing the production of new colon cells. But calcium has another role in that it combines with excess dietary fats to yield harmless soap-like compounds.[1] Of course, vitamin D is needed to help absorb calcium from the diet and make it available in the colon cells.

The antioxidant nutrients prevent the excess dietary fats and bile acids from oxidizing to form some of these harmful chemicals. Dietary fiber increases peristalsis, which moves the materials in the bowel along faster, but dietary fiber also plays another important role in providing the food for the "good" bacteria in the intestine to live on. If the good bacteria are thriving, then the "bad" bacteria are crowded out. The bad bacteria are what produce these harmful chemicals when they die and decompose.

Dietary fiber is not *digested* by us; that's why it used to be called "roughage." However, the good bacteria in our bowels do digest this fiber that we can't, and they feed and grow on it. The better the good bacteria grow, the harder it is for the bad bacteria to multiply.

You can see that the harmful chemicals—whether they come from dead bacteria, dietary fat, bile or whatever—are the biggest part of the problem. There is much that we can do to prevent them from causing colon cancer, however. Dietary fiber, antioxidant nutrients, calcium and fats all have a role. I will explain more about the harmful chemicals and the protective roles of the nutrients, but if you are not interested in more details, just skip ahead to the discussion on using supplements to reduce your risk of colon cancer.

Fecapentaenes

Scientists have isolated the compounds produced by the decaying substances that can cause colon cancer.[2-5] These compounds, which are conjugated ether pentaenyl lipids, are called fecapentaenes for short. There are about twenty fecapentaenes that can mutate colon cells.

Most people consider bacteria as "germs." The fact is that some bacteria are pathogenic, i.e., they cause disease, and some are not. In fact, we are dependent on the "good" bacteria in our intestines. They produce nutrients such as biotin, folic acid, and vitamin B12, and they convert some of the food that we can't digest into nutri- ents that we can use, such as short-chain fatty acids.

There is a close relationship between health and the type of bacteria we have in our colon. When "good" bacteria are in short supply in the colon, it becomes dominated by putrefactive bacteria which generate toxins.

People who eat a high-fiber diet have mostly good bacteria [*Lactobacillus acidophilus, Lactobacillus bulgaricus, Lactobacillus bifidum (Bifidobacterium bifidus)*, and *Bifidobacterium longum*], while those eating low-fiber diets harbor mostly the "bad" bacteria (the patho- genic strains of bifidobacteria and bacteroides). *The good bacteria do not decompose bile, fats, and other chemicals into compounds that cause cancer, whereas the bad bacteria do. Nor do the good bacteria themselves decompose into harmful compounds, whereas the bad bacteria do.*

The Finns, who eat a high-fat, high-fiber diet, and also eat ample amounts of yogurt, have a relatively low incidence of colon cancer. They have been shown to harbor large numbers of good bacteria such as the *Lactobacillus bulgaricus* from yogurt in their intestines.

Clinical studies have shown that those persons consuming dietary supplements of *Lactobacillus acidophilus* daily have greatly diminished levels of the enzymes that produce the harmful decomposition products. In laboratory animal studies where carcinogens were given to rats fed large amounts of *Lactobacillus acidophilus,* the colon cancer incidence was much lower than in those not protected by the good bacteria.

Bile

Bile is produced by the liver to help in the digestion of fats. Bile is stored in the gallbladder until it is needed in the duodenum portion of the small intestine to emulsify fats to make them digest better. The more fat that is eaten, the more bile that is produced and emptied into the intestine.

The two main components of bile are cholic acid and deoxy-cholic acid. If the bile is allowed to stagnate in the bowel for a long period, some types of bacteria will convert the cholic acid into another proven cancer-causer, apcholic acid; the deoxycholic acid will be converted into 3-methyl-cholanthrene (3-MCA), one of the most dangerous cancer producers known.

It's obvious that we don't want a sluggish bowel that allows time for bile decomposition products to be in contact with the colon walls for extended periods of time. Nor do we want high-fat diets that increase the production of bile.

Fiber

The health-food community has stressed the need for "roughage" and "bulk" since its inception. Few established nutritionists or physicians listened. They sought to reassure Americans that their highly refined diet was just great and that there was no need for "daily regularity."

It wasn't until the early 1970s that Drs. Dennis P. Burkitt and H. C. Trowel published their epidemiological studies linking low-fiber intake to the high incidence of colon cancer, coronary heart disease, obesity, diabetes, hypertension, constipation, gall stones, irritable colon, appendicitis, hemorrhoids, hiatus hernia, and diverticular diseases of the colon among Western people.[6,7] Indeed, previously, the preferred treatment for many of these disorders included being placed on a refined, bland diet.

In 1980, the British Royal College of Physicians recommended an increased consumption of fiber. In 1983, the British Health Education Council suggested that dietary fiber be increased by 50 percent. In 1985, the U.S. National Cancer Institute (NCI) advised that the optimal fiber intake is about 25 to 35 grams per day. This fits in nicely with the 25/25 diet I discussed in the preceding chapter on breast cancer. The 25/25 diet is a practical diet where no more than 25 *percent* of calories are obtained from fat and there are at least 25 *grams* of fiber in the diet. (One ounce equals about 28 grams.) In 1986, the NCI recommended that Americans double the amount of fiber they eat. (They really meant for the average American to double the dietary fiber—some of us were already eating enough fiber.)

Even with all the studies, many physicians and scientists were still not convinced. When a food company introduced a high-fiber cereal that stated on its package that some cancers, and in particular, colon cancer, were related to diet, the regulatory agencies had conniptions. They were forced to remove the information—the same information that the NCI was trying to get to the public.

Since the Burkitt and Trowel studies, several laboratory animal, epidemiological and clinical studies have confirmed the link of a low-fiber diet with a higher incidence of colon cancer. This information has been summarized by Dr. David Kritchevsky of the Wistar Institute. The U.S. Food and Drug Administration contracted the Life Sciences Research Office of the Federation of American Societies For Experimental Medicine to compile and analyze the data, which Dr. Kritchevsky published.

As mentioned earlier, fiber stimulates the bowel muscles to move the bowel contents along. A high-fiber diet normally produces a transit time through the body of one to two days. The food consumed by Africans eating their normal tribal diets in the Burkitt and Trowell studies, traveled from mouth through the body in one day. In contrast, the food consumed by the average Westerner (high in fat and low in fiber) requires at least three days for the same trip. Indeed, many low-fiber diets require up to two weeks to be passed through the system.

The high-fiber diet of the Africans contains about 25 grams of fiber daily. The average Western diet contains only about 8 grams daily. The difference is an average of about three-quaarters of an ounce daily. In a meta-analysis of thirteen other studies of dietary fiber and colon cancer, researchers at the University of Toronto estimate that if the average person adds 13 grams of fiber to his or her daily diet, the overall incidence of colon cancer would be reduced by about 30 percent.[8]

Those who eat low-fiber diets not only tend to have bac-

**teria that produce cancer-causing chemicals but also have a
slow transit time that keeps these chemicals concentrated
and in contact with their bowel for long periods.**

High-fiber diets also have a diluting action. The larger volume
of fiber dilutes the cancer-causing chemicals to reduce their odds
of being transported through the colon cell walls. The Finns, who
eat a high-fat, high-fiber diet that produces three times the fecal
bulk of Americans, have only one-third the colon cancer incidence
of the U.S.

High-fiber diets, rich in wheat bran or cellulose, reduce colon
cancer risk by lowering the production of fecapentaenes, secondary
bile acids and other mutagens.[9] Confirming studies indicate that
wheat bran may be the most effective fiber for preventing colorectal cancer.[10]

If you don't wish to count daily grams of fiber, there are two
good rules of thumb that may help you. Eat enough fiber until
you notice that your stools float and have the consistency of a ripe
banana (peeled, of course) and your transit time is about two days
or less. Transit time can be measured by noting how long it takes
for a "spike" of powdered charcoal to appear as a black mark in
your stools. Suitable powdered charcoal is available in most health
food and drug stores as an aid for "gas."

As discussed earlier, fiber is the part of food that is not digested
in the small intestine. Fiber is classified into two groups, soluble
or insoluble. There are five main classes of fiber: cellulose, hemicel-
lulose, gum, pectin and lignin.

Each class has a different effect on bowel health, so you should
have ample amounts of each in your diet. The type of fiber influences water retention and stool softness, the bacteria population
(different bacteria feed on different foods), and the dry bulk which
consists of the fiber plus the bacteria. Insoluble fiber offers the best
protection against colon cancer, while soluble fiber helps protect
against heart disease.

Vegetables, whole wheat, and most whole grains have a fiber
content that is mostly insoluble. Fruits, oats, barley and legumes
have a fiber content that is mostly soluble. Oat bran and beans are
especially good sources of soluble fiber. Guar gum, oat bran and

vegetable fiber are excellent supplements that can be added to your favorite foods, mixed in juices, or chewed as tablets.

Keep in mind that the more natural or "whole" the foods are in the diet, the better your odds of having all five fiber classes working for your health. Conversely, the more refined or fractionated your food products are, the lower your diet will be in all classes of fiber.

Calcium and Vitamin D

I discussed the protective roles of calcium and vitamin D in Chapter 14, and the interesting serendipitous manner in which its protective role was discovered. Now I will present a few specifics.

Calcium is needed for the normal progression of growth and reproduction of the epithelial cells that line the colon. If calcium is lacking, the cells grow abnormally. Increased dietary calcium inhibits the hyperproliferation of colon epithelial cells that is common to high-risk persons. In high-risk persons, a protective effect is observed at dietary calcium levels above 1,500 milligrams daily.[11-14]

A 15-year case control study in Sweden has confirmed that a high intake of calcium and cereal fiber reduced the risk of colon cancer.[15]

The Antioxidant Nutrients

There are several mechanisms by which the antioxidants protect against colon cancer; some protect the intestinal cells themselves, others prevent free-radical reactions from rendering the bowel contents carcinogenic.

Italian researchers fed high-risk patients supplements of vitamins A, C and E, and found that these supplements were effective in reducing abnormalities in cell kinetics that are involved in precancerous conditions.[16]

Researchers at the University of Toronto fed colon cancer patients vitamin C and E supplements after surgery and studied them after two years. They concluded that vitamins C and E reduced polyp recurrence by 20 percent.[17]

Harvard's Dr. Walter C. Willett also participated in a research project that included many researchers from several organizations. They found that vitamin E, as measured in the blood, was inversely related to the risk of colorectal cancer. They believe the risk reduction is modest, and they recommend further studies.[18]

Several laboratory animal studies have shown selenium protective against chemical-carcinogen-induced colon cancer.[19] A case-control study of risk factors of colorectal cancer was conducted in China and Yugoslavia, and blood selenium levels were found to be significantly lower in colon cancer patients.[20,21] A Polish study also found that blood levels of selenium were significantly lower in gastrointestinal cancer patients.[22]

Exercise

Inactivity or lack of exercise is a risk factor in all of the cancers in which dietary fat and/or body fat are risk factors. This is primarily because inactivity leads to increased body fat. Some researchers believe that combining a high-fat diet with inactivity accounts for as much as 60 percent of all colorectal cancers for men, and 40 percent of all colorectal cancers for women.[23,24]

Polyps

Polyps themselves are not harmful, but many physicians feel that polyps, over time, have a high probability of turning into a malignant tumor. Therefore, most physicians prefer to remove polyps so that there is no chance they could become a problem later.

If you have a history of polyps, or a family history of polyps or colon cancer, then you should pay close attention to colon cancer risk factors, and follow a low-fat, high-fiber, high-antioxidant diet without fail.

Smoking

Smokers have twice the risk of colon polyps that nonsmokers do, and when the number of cigarettes smoked is examined, the increased risk is linear up to two-pack-a-day smokers, who have six times the risk of nonsmokers. This increased risk for polyps may be linked to smoking's interaction with vitamin C. Smokers have less available vitamin C in their bodies, even when they consume as much of the vitamin as nonsmokers. However, the link to colon cancer directly seems to be a weak, 10-percent increase in risk.

Alcohol

The relationship between alcohol consumption and colorectal cancer was examined in 52 studies between 1957 and 1991, with an association or increased risk found in most. The alcoholic beverage producing the strongest link to colon cancer is beer.[25,26] The highest risk is among those drinking more than 42 cans of beer a month. There are several ways that alcohol can interact, including promotion of carcinogens and stimulation of mucosal cell proliferation. Beer may contain nitrosamines or other unabsorbed carcinogens or precarcinogens that are activated in the intestine.

Prevention and Treatment

If you are concerned about colorectal cancer, you may wish to follow the 25/25 diet described earlier, which is a moderate-fat, moderate-fiber diet. Needless to say, the good life-style habits of exercising, not smoking, and moderate or no drinking will help. However, the following supplements are extremely important.

NUTRIENT	DAILY QUANTITY
calcium	1,000-1,500 mg
vitamin D	400 IU
L. acidophilus, L. bulgaricus, B. longum	2-3 capsules
vitamin E	200-600 IU
vitamin C	1,250-12,000 mg
selenium	200 mcg
beta-carotene	10,000-20,000 IU
pycnogenol	30 mg
bran	10 grams
garlic	1-3 capsules
fish oil	1 capsule
zinc	10-15 mg

At this writing, the five-year "cure" rate for colorectal cancer is about 53 percent. Hopefully, it will improve. The prudent approach is to contact the Cancer Information Service at 1-800-4-CANCER and see what the best treatments are at this time. Follow up the conventional treatment with shark cartilage therapy.

REFERENCES

1. G. V. Appleton, R. W. Owen, and R. C. Williamson, "The effect of dietary calcium supplementation on intestinal lipid metabolism," *Journal of Steroid Biochemistry and Molecular Biology* (May, 1992) 42(3-4):383-7.
2. A. C. Povey et al., "Laboratory and epidemiological studies of fecapentaenes," *Mutation Research* (March/April, 1991) 259(3-4):387-97.
3. C. E. Voogd et al., "Structure, chemical reactivity, and in vitro mutagenic activity in a series of fecapentaene analogues," *Mutant. Res.* (March, 1990) 243(3):195-9.
4. L. B. Vertegaal et al., "Further studies on the mutagenic activity of fecapentaene-12 analogues and conclusions about their molecular mode of action," *Mutat. Res.* (Feb. 1992) 281(2):93-8.
5. J. H. Weisburger et al., "Carcinogenicity tests of fecapentaene-12 in mice and rats," *Cancer Letters* (Feb. 1990) 49(2):89-98.

6. D. P. Burkitt, "Epidemiology of cancer of the colon and rectum," *Cancer* (1971) 28:3-12.

7. D. P. Burkitt, "Some diseases characteristic of modern Western civilization," *British Medical Journal* (1973) 1:274-8.

8. G. R. Howe et al., "Dietary intake of fiber and decreased risk of cancers of the colon and rectum: Evidence from the combined analysis of 13 case-control studies," *Journal of the National Cancer Institute* (Dec. 16, 1992) 84(24):1851-3.

9. B. Reddy et al. "The effects of types of fiber on neutral sterols in healthy subjects," *Cancer Research* (1989) 49:4629-35.

10. D. Albets et al., "Effects of dietary wheat-bran fiber on rectal epithelial cell proliferation in patients with resection for colorectal cancers." *J. Nat'l Cancer Inst.* (1990) 82:1280-5.

11. H. L. Newmark and M. Lipkin, "Calcium, vitamin D and colon cancer," *Cancer Research* (April 1, 1992) 52 (7 Suppl):2067s-2070s.

12. G. H. Barsoum et al., "Reduction of mucosal crypt cell proliferation in patients with colorectal adenomatous polyps by dietary calcium supplementation," *British Journal of Surgery* (June 1992) 79(6):581-3.

13. G. Arbman et al., "Cereal fiber, calcium and colorectal cancer," *Cancer* (April 15, 1992) 69(8):2042-8.

14. P. Rozen et al., "Oral calcium supplements suppress increased rectal epithelial proliferation of persons at risk of colorectal cancer," *Gut* (1989) 30:650-5.

15. M. J. Wargovich et al., "Calcium supplementation decreases rectal epithelial cell proliferation in subjects with sporadic adenoma," *Gastroenterology* (July 1992) 103(1):92-7.

16. G. M. Paganelli et al., "Effect of vitamin A, C, and E supplementation on rectal cell proliferation in patients with colorectal adenomas," *J. Nat'l Cancer Inst.* (Jan. 1, 1992) 84(1)47-51.

17. G. McKeown-Eyssen et al., "A randomized trial of vitamin C and vitamin E. supplementation in the prevention and recurrence of colorectal polyps," *Preventive Medicine* (1987) 16:275.

18. M. P. Longnecker et al., "Serum alpha-tocopherol concentration in relation to subsequent colorectal cancer: Pooled data from five cohorts, *J. Nat'l. Cancer Inst.* (March 18, 1992) 84(6):430-5.

19. M. M. Jacobs, C. F. Forst and F. A. Beams, "Biochemical and clinical effects of selenium on dimethylhydrazine-induced colon cancer in rats," *Cancer Res.* (Nov. 1981) 41(11):4458-65.

20. N. Zhao, "A case-control study of risk factors of colorectal cancer

in Shanxi Province," *Chung Hua Liu Hsing Ping Hsueh Tsa Chih* (Oct. 1990) 11(5):295-8.

21. M. Mikac-Devic, N. Vukelic and K. Kljaic, "Serum selenium level in patients with colorectal cancer," *Biological Trace Element Research* (April-June 1992) 33:87-94.

22. Z. Pawlowicz et al., "Blood selenium concentrations and glutathione peroxidase activities in patients with breast cancer and with advanced gastrointestinal cancer," *J. Trace Elem. Electrolytes Health Dis.* (Dec. 1991) 5(4):275-7.

23. A. Whittemore et al., "Diet, physical activity and colorectal cancer among Chinese in North America and China," *J. Nat. Cancer Inst.* (1990) 82:915-26.

24. M. Slatterly et al., "Physical activity, diet, and the risk for colon cancer in Utah," *American Journal of Epidemiology* (1987) 126:766.

25. G. A. Kune and L. Vitetta, "Alcohol consumption and the etiology of colorectal cancer: A review of the scientific evidence from 1957 to 1991," *Nutrition and Cancer* (1992) 18(2):97-111.

26. James E. Enstrom, "Colorectal cancer and beer drinking," *British Journal of Cancer* (1977) 35:674-83.

CHAPTER 21

Skin Cancer

One third of all cancers in the U.S. are skin cancers. Like most cancers, skin cancer is something we can do a lot about! We can take individual measures, and collectively, as the temporary inhabitants of this planet, we can stop the pollution that is destroying the protective ozone layer.

At one time, it was very fashionable for Caucasians to *look* healthy and beautiful by sporting deep suntans. I agree, it looks good while it lasts, but sun exposure hastens wrinkling later on. It was even a status symbol for blacks, who thought that they were naturally protected, to bake in the sun to demonstrate that they had leisure time. I agree, it felt good. However, excess ultraviolet energy from the sun (and indoor tanning lamps) immediately depressed the immune system of sun worshippers and damaged their skin in such a way that the results didn't show up for twenty years. Many who used sunscreens and/or took antioxidant nutrients were probably sufficiently protected to avoid skin cancer. Many of the others are part of the statistics.

In 1991, there were more than 500,000 new cases of basal cell carcinoma, more than 100,000 new cases of squamous cell carcinoma, and more than 32,000 new cases of malignant melanoma.

Malignant melanoma, the most deadly form of cancer, is increasing at a rapid rate. The chances of getting malignant melanoma were one in 1,500 in 1930, one in 250 in 1980, one in 135 in 1987, and in 1993, the estimate for the year 2000 is a shocking one

166

in 90. In 1980, there were 14,000 cases of malignant melanoma in the U.S. The estimate for the year 2000 is 37,000. In 1992, about 6,700 persons died of malignant melanoma.

The 1993 estimates for the less serious forms of skin cancer, basal cell and squamous cell carcinoma, are that one or the other will develop in three in ten adults during their lifetimes. For those born after 1985, the estimate is that four in ten will develop either basal cell or squamous cell carcinoma.

About thirty laboratories around the world are studying the effect of excess ultraviolet (UV) energy on the immune system. The meaning of this effect is not clearly understood at this writing, but it is believed that some sunlight stimulates the immune system. Even sunshine reaching the retina produces a good healthy response, and it helps relieve depression. But, as we know that *too much* UV reaching the eyes can cause cataracts, *too much* UV can depress the immune system.

Dr. Mark Green of the Harvard Medical School has discovered that *excess* UV selectively neutralizes cells that are important in activating immune responses. These are the antibody presenting cells that reside in the skin, spleen and other organs throughout the body. They help control the body's defense against invaders by recognizing them and summoning white blood cells (lymphocytes) to destroy the intruders.

In Australia, a team of researchers led by Dr. Peter Hersey found that volunteers who tanned for 30 minutes daily for 12 days in a commercial tanning salon had two measurable changes to their immune systems. They had an increase in suppressor cells, which turn off some immune responses, and a decrease in helper cells. These abnormalities *persisted* for more than two weeks after the exposure to the UV.

Remember, UV doesn't affect the skin only—it reaches the blood circulating through the skin, and can affect many blood components. It can destroy vitamins, generate free radicals and harm immune system components, regardless of our skin pigmentation!

Your first line of defense is to moderate your sun exposure. It is not just the amount of time you sunbathe, but the cumulative time your face, hands, neck, etc. are exposed to daylight. Your second line of defense is to take the antioxidant nutrients that minimize free-radical damage. Your third line of defense is to encourage the reduction of production and release of the chloro-fluorocarbons and other gases that destroy our protective ozone layer in the stratosphere. Ozone absorbs much of the UV energy from the sun, but recent depletions of the protective ozone layer have resulted in more than twice as much UV energy reaching the ground. This has an effect on most living things, not just human skin cancers.

Antioxidant Nutrients

Many laboratory animal studies have shown that selenium is very protective against UV. In fact, when selenium first became available as a food supplement, many people complained to me that they didn't tan as readily. They came back from their vacations with little tan. I had recommended selenium to them to protect them against sunburn, which is important to me. Selenium is protective against sunburn during exposure, and even limits the development of the redness after your exposure. That redness is a result of continuing free-radical reactions.

Researchers often use a strain of mice that are hairless in laboratory studies of antioxidants' protection against skin cancer. These studies consistently find a very strong protective effect against UV-induced skin damage and cancer and even chemical carcinogen-induced skin cancer.[1-3]

In Chapter 10, on selenium, I discussed the study in which Dr. Larry Clark and colleagues at Cornell determined the blood selenium levels in 240 skin cancer patients and compared the results to those from 103 apparently healthy persons living in low-selenium areas. The mean blood-selenium level for the skin cancer patients was significantly lower than that of the apparently healthy individuals. After adjusting for age, sun damage to the skin, blood beta-carotene and vitamin A levels, and other factors, the incidence of skin cancer in those persons in the lowest tenth of blood selenium levels was 5.8 times as great as those in the top tenth.[3]

It should be noted that selenium, in the form of the common food supplement L-selenomethionine, can protect skin against sun-induced damage.[4] Beta-carotene, other carotenoids and vitamin A are very protective against skin cancer development and skin cancer spread as well.[5,6]

Dr. Helen Gensler of the University of Arizona college of Medicine and Cancer Center has found that rubbing vitamin E on the skin "drastically cuts skin cancer risk." It is not just a matter of the vitamin E protecting the skin, but a matter of vitamin E protecting the immune response. In an experiment in which mice were exposed to a very large amount of UV energy, only 42 percent of the vitamin-E treated animals developed cancer, compared to 81 percent of the untreated mice.[7] The analysis of splenocytes revealed that the vitamin E treatment prevented UV-induced suppression of immunity.[7]

Remember, vitamin E doesn't build up quickly in the skin. It takes several weeks to build up skin tissue to a protective amount. You can't just take your first vitamin E capsule and run out into the sunshine thinking that you are protected.

Prevention

Needless to say, moderating your exposure to sunlight is most important. Using a sunscreen and wide-brimmed hats are prudent measures. A side benefit is that your skin will look ten to fifteen years younger than your friends' of your same age who don't protect themselves against sun damage.

You may also wish to consider taking the following food supplements.

NUTRIENT	DAILY AMOUNT
selenium	200 mcg
vitamin E	200-600 IU

NUTRIENT (con't)	DAILY AMOUNT
beta-carotene	10,000-15,000 IU
vitamin A	5,000 IU
vitamin C	1,000-11,000 mg
pycnogenol	30-60 mg
evening primrose oil	one capsule

REFERENCES

1. K. Overad et al., "Selenium inhibits UV-light-induced skin carcino-genesis in hairless mice," *Cancer Letters* (1985) 27(2):163-170.
2. M. P. Bansal and G. Gupta, "Influence of selenium on 3-methylcholanthrene induced skin carcinogenesis in mice," *Journal of Environmental Pathology, Toxicology and Oncology* (1988) 8(7):49-53.
3. L. C. Clark et al., "Plasma selenium and skin neoplasms: A case-controlled study," *Nutrition & Cancer* (Jan.–March 1984) 6(1):13-21.
4. Karen E. Burke, "Skin cancer protection with L. selenomethionine," *Nutr. Rept.* (Oct., 1992) 10(10):73,80.
5. J. J. DeCosse, "Potential for chemoprevention," *Cancer* (1982) 50(11):2550-53.
6. G. L. Peck, "Chemoprevention of cancer with retinoids," *Gynecological Oncology* (1981) 12(2):S331-40.
7. H. Gensler and M. Magdaleno, "Topical vitamin E inhibition of im-munosuppression and tumorigenesis induced by ultraviolet irradia-tion," *Nutrition & Cancer* (1991) 15:97-106.

CHAPTER 22

Prostate Cancer

Prostate cancer is somewhat analogous to breast cancer. Although men can have breast cancer, women can't have prostate cancer. Aside from that, when lung cancer incidence falls, as it should, prostate cancer will be the leading cancer in men and breast cancer will be the leading cancer in women. Statistically, 103 men in a thousand will develop prostate cancer, while 110 women will develop breast cancer according to 1992 figures.

We already have enough knowledge to virtually eliminate lung cancer, and greatly reduce breast cancer, but we still have too much to learn about prostate cancer to say with certainty that we can reduce its incidence drastically.

There is a significant free-radical involvement, thus the antioxidant nutrients will have a significant effect. Also, looking at cancer incidence maps such as those in Chapter 14, it is apparent that sunshine and vitamin D have a protective effect.

In 1993, about 132,000 men were newly diagnosed as having prostate cancer and about 34,000 men died of it. The incidence rate has increased by 39 percent since 1973.

The healthy prostate gland weighs about an ounce and is a walnut- or olive-size gland that surrounds the urethra at the base of the bladder. Due to its location, it can be readily examined by a physician digitally through the rectum for enlargement and tumors. The function of the prostate gland is to make the seminal fluid that is added to semen for ejaculation.

Men are prone to have an enlargement of the prostate that interferes with urination as they age. However, there is an extremely strong dietary component for the benign prostate enlargement called benign prostatic hypertrophy (BPH). Dietary deficiencies of zinc and omega-3 fatty acids such as those found in fish oils are linked to BPH. Another disorder of the prostate is prostatitis. These disorders of the prostate are not malignant, and are discussed more fully in my book *The New Supernutrition*.[1]

If a man has difficulty urinating or needs to urinate frequently, he should immediately have his prostate examined and blood tests made. This is especially true if he has a family history of prostate cancer or is over the age of 55. It is important to catch prostate cancer before it spreads to the bones, which it can readily do.

There are two types of prostate cancers, one of which is very slow-growing, and the other very fast-growing. Unfortunately, it is impossible at this writing to tell which is which at first examination. The only way to tell is to watch, and then it is often too late if it turns out to be the fast-growing type.

Vasectomy

At this writing, two studies have indicated a slight link between vasectomies and prostate cancer, and five have shown no link. The two studies suggesting a slight link appear to be flawed.

Dietary Fat

The evidence is far from conclusive, but there may be a slight increase in risk of prostate cancer from a high-fat diet.[2-4] A study to examine the effect of a high-fat diet on the progression of prostate cancer found no effect.[5]

Body fat

The risk of prostate cancer does increase with increasing body fat. A moderately overweight man has a 2.3 times greater risk of prostate cancer and an obese (20 percent above normal) man has a four times greater risk.[6]

Smoking and Alcohol

At least one study shows that smokers have a significantly elevated risk—nearly twice (1.8x) the standard risk—for prostate cancer, but more studies are needed to make a firm conclusion.[7] So far, alcohol appears unrelated to risk.[7]

Vitamin A

The amount of vitamin A circulating in your blood is a significant factor in protection against prostate cancer. Researchers at the National Cancer Institute (NCI) and Johns Hopkins University drew blood samples in 1974 from 25,802 persons and followed their health for thirteen years. During that time 103 men developed prostate cancer.

When the blood samples were ranked in order of increasing levels of vitamin A, it was found that the men in the top half of vitamin A values had only 40 percent of the prostate cancer incidence of those in the lowest quarter.[8] Those in the third quarter had two-thirds the incidence of the lowest quarter.

In a similar but smaller study, also published in 1990, other researchers at the NCI examined the prostate cancer incidence in a group of 2,400 men who were healthy when they entered the study between 1971 and 1975. At the time the men entered the study, they had blood samples drawn. During ten years of follow-up, 84 men developed prostate cancer.

The blood samples were analyzed for those men and compared to other healthy men similarly matched in risk factors. The researchers found that when the blood vitamin A levels were ranked in increasing level of vitamin A that those men in the top quarter had only about 45 percent the prostate cancer incidence as those in the bottom quarter.[9] These two studies confirmed an earlier study.

Selenium

Selenium concentrates in the sex organs because it has several roles in both male and female sexual functions. As one example, selenium concentrates in the testes because selenium is an important component of sperm cells. Selenium also may have a role in prostaglandin production as the prostate contains appreciable amounts of selenium. A low selenium diet may contribute to both sterility and prostate disorders.[11]

Selenium inhibits the growth of human prostate carcinoma cells.[12] Another clue as to the protective effect of selenium is that cadmium is known to cause prostate cancer, and selenium protects against cadmium-induced prostate cancer.[13]

Fish Oils

Fish oils inhibit prostate cancer cells from growing when they are transplanted.[14] Researchers at Rutgers University, Memorial Sloan-Kettering Cancer Center and the American Health Foundation found that transplanted prostate tumor cells had reduced growth and more connective tissue than normal.

Preventing and Treating Prostate Cancer

At this writing there is an extremely critical difference in which procedure you choose for treatment. It is critical that the preferred treatment be used first, because if the standard treatment is used, then the newer and preferred treatment will not work. I'll discuss treatment shortly, but first let's consider prevention.

First of all, if you are over 50, don't rely merely on a digital rectal examination. You would want to catch any malignancy before drastic measures are required, especially if avoiding impotency is of interest. Yes, you need the annual anal exam, but you should also have blood tests for PSA and PAP taken yearly. (That's a Prostatic Acid Phosphatase (PAP) blood test, not a "Pap smear," which is, of course, the Papanicolaou test for precancerous cells in the cervix.) The Prostatic Specific Antigen (PSA) test measures the antigen which is made in, and only in, the prostate. PSA increases when the prostate is cancerous. This test is far superior to digital examination in catching prostate cancers before they have spread. If a cancer is detected while PSA is still in the range just above normal, fewer than a third of such cancers have spread. Digital exams, however, usually cannot detect the smaller tumors, and usually 70 percent have spread by the time they are detected digitally. The PSA test can give a positive reading four years ahead of the digital examination.

It is important to have regular PSA and PAP test made so that your baseline level is known. This can make a rise in PSA level more easily verified. The PSA test is not perfect. Sometimes it gives a false high reading—which needlessly frightens the patient—and sometimes it misses a cancer. But, when the PSA and PAP tests are combined with digital examination and ultrasound sonogram, the accuracy is very high. Most men with slightly elevated PSA levels do not have cancer, but another problem which can be clarified by other procedures, including biopsy.

You may wish to select the following supplements as part of your prostate cancer prevention program.

NUTRIENT	DAILY AMOUNT
vitamin A	5,000 IU
beta-carotene	15,000–25,000 IU
selenium	100–200 mcg
vitamin D	400 IU

NUTRIENT *(con't)*	DAILY AMOUNT
vitamin E	200-400 IU
vitamin C	1,000-12,500 mg
fish oils	4-8 capsules
zinc	25 mg
magnesium	200-400 mg

At this writing the standard treatments (which have been used since about 1950) are either radiation or the surgical removal of the tumor, followed by the surgical removal of the testicles and/or treatment with testosterone-lowering, estrogen-like drugs such as stilbestrol. The approach of lowering testosterone levels sounds prudent, but it is incomplete. A study published in 1982 in the *Journal of Urology* found that unfortunately, with this treatment patients fared no differently in terms of life-span, on the average, than with no treatment at all. Currently, the oncologists using the standard method are claiming a 60 to 80 percent "remission" rate.

Prostate tumors are androgen-dependent. Androgens are hormones that stimulate the development of male sex characteristics. The testes make androgens, but so do the adrenal glands, for which they were named. The conventional therapy does not affect the androgen production by the adrenals, and that is a fatal mistake. Dr. Fernand Labrie of Laval University in Quebec found that by using a drug called Lupron Depot (which interferes with luteinizing hormone-releasing hormone) along with the drug flutamide, androgen levels could be significantly lowered without castrating the patient, and *even advanced cases of prostate cancer that had spread to the bones could be cured*. At this writing, the success rate is above 95 percent with more than 800 patients.[16] *In addition, once the cancer is beaten, the drugs can be stopped and normal sexual function can be regained.*

It is important that the standard treatment not be used first, as the treatment appears to alter the cancer cells, and make the Labrie protocol ineffective. If you have already used the standard therapies, then you may wish to consider following up with shark cartilage therapy.

You can learn more about the Labrie protocol by contacting:

Lloyd Ney, Cancer Communications
PAACT Inc. (Patient Advocates for Advanced Cancer Treatments)
1143 Parmelee N.W.
Grand Rapids, Michigan 49504

PAACT is a nonprofit organization (in fact, it is the largest one of its type) dedicated to informing the public about the latest prostate cancer research, protocols and clinical studies. Donations are accepted in the form of memberships.

REFERENCES

1. Richard A. Passwater, *The New Supernutrition* (New York: Pocket Books, 1991).
2. A. B. Miller, "Diet and cancer: a review," *Acta Oncologica* (1990) 29(1):87-95.
3. B. E. Statland, "Nutrition and cancer," *Clinical Chemistry* (Aug., 1992) 38:1587-94.
4. L. N. Kolonel et al., "Role of diet in cancer incidence in Hawaii," *Cancer Research* (May, 1983) 43:2397s-2402s.
5. K. Takai, "Promotional effects of high-fat diet on chemical carcinogenesis of the prostate," *Nippon Hinyokika Gakkai Zasshi* (June, 1991) 82(6):871-80.
6. R. Talamini et al., "Nutrition, social factors and prostatic cancer in a Northern Italian population," *British Journal of Cancer* (1986) 53:817-21.
7. A. W. Hsing et al., "Diet, tobacco use, and fatal prostate cancer: results from the Lutheran Brotherhood Cohort Study," *Cancer Res.* (Nov. 1, 1990) 50(21):6836-40.
8. A. W. Hsing et al., "Serologic precursors of cancer: retinol, carotenoids, and tocopherol, and the risk of prostate cancer," *Journal of the National Cancer Institute* (June 6, 1990) 82(11):941-6.
9. M. E. Reichman, et al., "Serum vitamin A and subsequent development of prostate cancer in the first National Health and Nutrition Examination Survey Epidemiological Follow-up Study," *Cancer Res.* (Apr. 15, 1990) 50(8):3211-5.
10. R. B. Hayes et al., "Serum retinal and prostate cancer," *Cancer* (Nov. 1, 1988) 62(9):2021-6.
11. Richard A. Passwater, *Selenium as Food and Medicine* (New Canaan, CT: Keats Publishing, Inc., 1980).

12. M. M. Webber, E. A. Perez-Ripoll, G. T. James, "Inhibitory Effects of selenium on the growth of DU-145 human prostate carcinoma cells in vitro," *Biochemical and Biophysical Research Communications* (July 31, 1985) 130(2):603-9.

13. M. M. Webber, "Selenium prevents the growth stimulatory effects of cadmium on human prostatic epithelium," *Biochem. Biophys. Res. Commun.* (March 29, 1985) 127(3):871-7.

14. R. Karmah et al., "The effects of dietary omega-3 fatty acids on DU-145 transplantable human prostate tumors," *Antiox. Res.* (1987) 7:1173-9.

15. D. P. Rose and J. M. Connolly, "Dietary fat, fatty acids and prostate cancer," *Lipids* (Oct., 1992) 27(10):798-803.

16. Wayne Martin, "On prostate cancer," *Townsend Letter for Doctors* (Jan., 1992) 57-8.

CHAPTER 23

Cervical Cancer

Cervical cancer affects about 2 percent of American women, killing about 4,400 each year. The pre-invasive form is almost always curable, but once it becomes invasive, the cure rate drops to 50 percent. The good news is that early detection, thanks to the Pap smear (Papanicolaou test), has led to a 70 percent reduction in the death rate due to cervical cancer over the last 40 years.

Changes can occur in the surface cells of the uterine cervix that are premalignant—not yet cancer. This condition is called cervical dysplasia or cervical intraepithelial neoplasia or carcinoma *in situ*. This condition, if left untreated, may turn into cervical cancer. The good news is that vitamin C and folic acid supplements can readily convert these cells back to normal cells, thus avoiding the development of cervical cancer.

This is the most common concern of women who have their annual Pap smear. There are other, more troublesome, cures as well, but women can save themselves a lot of worry and expense if they get adequate vitamin C and folic acid.

Risk factors that enhance the progress of cervical dysplasia towards cervical cancer include women who became sexually active before the age of 18, have had multiple sex partners, or their partners have had multiple partners.

The sexual transmission of the human papillomavirus (HPV) is a co-carcinogen. *The presence of HPV increases a woman's risk by 2,000 times.* About 80 percent of all cervical cancers are caused by

HPV. How does a woman obtain this not-so-friendly virus? from sex with a male who has the virus. Of course, the more men she has sex with, the more chances she has of finding one carrying the virus. Naturally, the more partners the male has had, the greater the chance that he will have the HPV virus.

There are about 60 different HPV ranging from the less dangerous kinds that cause genital warts and plantar warts, to the co-carcinogenic HPV-16 and HPV-18. When HPV-16 infects the cervix, a nearly invisible flat wart occurs. But sex hormones such as progesterone transform these warts into wildly growing cancer cells. Thus, HPV-16 and progesterone are a deadly team.[1] A deficiency of folate (folic acid) makes matters even worse, as the deficiency facilitates invasion of the virus.

Contraceptives, including condoms, diaphragms, foams and spermicidal jellies or creams, are all fairly effective in blocking the transmission of HPV. Their proper use reduces HPV transmission by about 75 percent.

Oral Contraceptive Use and Risk

Women who use oral contraceptives have less folate (folic acid, a member of the vitamin B-complex family, although it is not a vitamin) in their cervical cells—but not necessarily in their blood—than those women who eat the same diet but do not take "the pill." This decrease in cervical cell folate leads to cervical dysplasia, which is reversed with increased folate.[2]

It is not known why oral contraceptives lower the amount of folate in cervical cells, but it may be due to influence of sex hormones on cervical tissue. The main point is that this is an important observation because folate protects the cervix from dysplasia by preventing HPV invasion.

One study shows that women who have cervical dysplasia have increased risk of cervical cancer when they take the pill. Other women do not have this increased risk with the pill. The researchers also found that women who had dysplasia and took the pill had an apparent improvement at first, which disappeared after two years and was followed by cervical cancer.

A 1992 study by Dr. A. M. Kaunitz of the University of Florida concluded that the most recent statistical evidence confirms a protective effect of oral contraceptive use against *ovarian and endometrial* cancer, but the relationship to cervical cancer was too hampered by confounding factors.[3]

The problem of confounding factors may have been resolved with a meta-analysis of 21 studies. Oral contraceptives were associated with increased risk of 50 percent for cervical dysplasia, and 20 percent for cervical cancer.[4]

There is the possibility that the newer birth control pills are safer.

Smoking and Risk

There is a weak link between smoking and cervical cancer. According to one study, women who smoke a pack a day for more than 12 years have 12 times the risk of developing cervical cancer. Another study finds that "light smokers" have twice (2.2x) the risk, and "heavy smokers" have four (3.9) times the risk.[5] Yet another study found only a small increase in risk for all women, which disappeared when controlled for other confounding factors.[6] However, when this study considered only the women, both smokers and nonsmokers, who were infected with HPV-16 or HPV-18, the smokers had five times the risk.

No link has been established between alcohol and cervical cancer.[5]

Douching and Risk

Douching with anything but water or water plus vinegar increases the risk of cervical cancer. Women who douche more than once a week have four times the risk than those who douche less often have.[7]

Folate

I have mentioned that folate prevents the invasion of HPV into the cells. This information comes from the many years of research by Dr. Charles E. Butterworth, Jr. and his colleagues. Dr. Butterworth first reported in 1980 that a folate deficiency was associated with increased cervical dysplasia and that it could be reversed with folate supplementation.[8] He eventually tracked down the reason to be that the folate deficiency facilitates the incorporation of HPV into the DNA of cervical cells.[9,10] The HPV the "captures" the DNA and forces it to manufacture more HPV, and the invasion begins.

Antioxidant Nutrients

In addition to folate, three antioxidant nutrients play an important role in preventing cervical dysplasia and cervical cancer; vitamin C, vitamin E and beta-carotene.[11-16] Moderate deficiency of each alone doubles the risk of cervical dysplasia. Severe deficiency of each alone triples the risk.

Selenium was also found to be protective against both cervical dysplasia and cervical cancer.[17-19]

Prevention and Treatment

I have already discussed prevention: a simple yearly Pap smear for early detection, and generous amounts of folate (folic acid) and the antioxidant nutrients.

NUTRIENT	DAILY AMOUNT
folate (folic acid)	800 mcg-3 mg
vitamin C	1,250-11,000 mg
vitamin A	5,000 IU
beta-carotene	10,000-25,000 IU
vitamin E	200-600 IU
selenium	200 mcg

As for the treatment, the standard procedures are very effective if used early. And since cervical cancer is normally slow growing, there is no good reason not to detect it early with Pap smears.

If the cancer is advanced, the standard treatments are still 50 percent effective. Following standard treatment with shark cartilage treatment is recommended at this time. Check with the cancer information sources listed in Chapter 17 for the latest information.

REFERENCES

1. "Deadly duo leads to cancer of the cervix," *Science News* (Jan. 1993) 143:38.
2. N. Whitehead et al., "Megaloblastic changes in the cervical epithelium: Association with oral contraceptive therapy and reversal with folic acid," *Journal of the American Medical Association* (1973) 226:1421-4.
3. A. M. Kaunitz, "Oral contraceptives and gynecological cancer: An update for the 1990s," *American Journal of Obstetrics and Gynecology* (Oct. 1992) 167(4):1171-6.
4. M. Delgado-Rodriguez et al., "Oral contraceptives and cancer of the cervix uteri: A meta-analysis," *Acta Obstetricia et Gynecologica Scandinavica* (July 1992) 71(5):368-76.
5. J. C. Licciardone et al., "Cigarette smoking and alcohol consumption in the aetiology of uterine cervical cancer," *International Journal of Epidemiology* (Sept. 1989) 18(3):533-7.
6. R. Herrero et al., "Invasive cervical cancer and smoking in Latin America," *Journal of the National Cancer Institute* (Feb. 1, 1989) 81(3):205-11.
7. John W. Gardner et al., *American Journal of Epidemiology* (Feb. 15, 1992).
8. Charles E. Butterworth, Jr. et al., "Folate-induce regression of cervical intraepithelial neoplasia in users of oral contraceptive agents," *American Journal of Clinical Nutrition* (1980) 33:926.
9. Charles E. Butterworth, Jr. "Effect of folate on cervical cancer: synergism among risk factors," *Annals of the New York Academy of Sciences* (Sept. 30, 1992) 669:293-9.
10. P. Fekete and A. Hammani, "Folic acid-like deficiency in cervicovaginal smears: a possible manifestation of papillomavirus infection," *Acta Cytologica* (1987) 31:697.

11. D. I. Buckley et al., "Dietary micronutrients and cervical dysplasia in southwestern American Indian women," *Nutrition and Cancer* (1992) 17(2):179-85.
12. R. Herrero et al., "A case-control study of nutrient status and invasive cervical cancer: I. dietary indicators," *Amer. J. Epidemiol.* (Dec. 1, 1991) 134(11):1335-46.
13. J. W. Orr et al., "Nutritional status of patients with untreated cervical cancer: II. vitamin assessment," *Amer. J. Obstet. Gynecol.* (March 1, 1985) 151(5):632-5.
14. K. E. Brock et al., "Nutrients in the diet and plasma and risk of in situ cervical cancer," *J. Natl. Cancer Inst.* (June 15, 1988) 80(8):580-5.
15. S. Wassertheil-Smoller et al., "Dietary vitamin C and uterine cervical dysplasia," *Amer. J. Epidemiol.* (Nov. 1981) 114(5):714-24.
16. R. Verreault et al., "A case-control study of diet and invasive cervical cancer," *International Journal of Cancer* (1989) 43:1050-4.
17. M. L. Slattery et al., "Dietary vitamins A, C, and E and selenium as risk factors for cervical cancer," *Epidemiology* (Jan. 1990) 1(1):8-15.
18. K. E. Brock et al., "Serum selenium level in relation to in situ cervical cancer in Australia," *J. Natl. Cancer Inst.* (Feb. 20, 1991) 83(4):292-3.
19. H. Sundstrom, O. Ylikorkala and A. Kauppila, "Serum selenium and thromboxane in patients with gynaecological cancer," *Carcinogenesis* (July 1986) 7(7):1051-2.

APPENDIX A

The Immune System

This information is reprinted from Selenium as Food and Medicine *for the benefit of those wishing to understand what the immune system entails and how nutrients play a role in stimulating the production of various components of this vital system.*[1]

The body protects itself against invasion by disease microorganisms through its ability to recognize itself and to reject and destroy everything that is non-self. The mechanism that accomplishes this is the immune system. As Dr. Robert Good of the Sloan-Kettering Institute for Cancer Research puts it, "Man lives in a sea of micro-organisms; the immune system is his license to survive."[2]

The immune system is a complex network of lymphocytes (white blood cells formed in the lymph tissue), macrophages (large, scavenger white blood cells), antibodies (proteins that can react with specific germs) and interferon (an anti-viral and anti-tumor compound).

The immune system produces three types of lymphocytes called T-cells, B-cells and K-cells. The T-cells have the ability to reject all foreign matter, while B-cells have the ability to produce antibodies. Relatively little is understood about the T-cells and B-cells, but still less is known about the "killer" K-cells which are involved in an immune phenomenon called *antibody-dependent cell-mediated cytotoxicity.*

Schematic showing the major components of the immune system

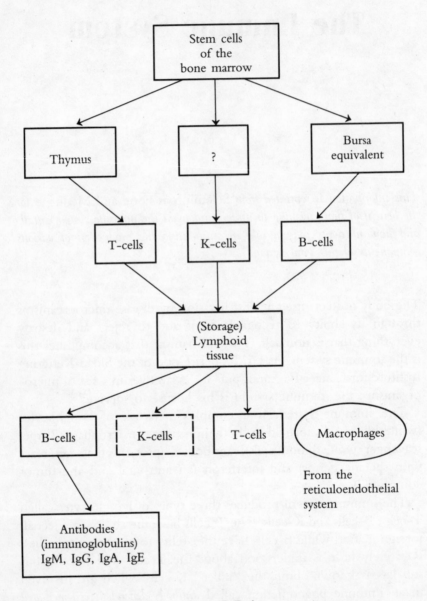

FIGURE A.

All three specialized lymphocytes are formed from the same basic cell of the bone marrow called a stem cell. The figure at left illustrates how stem cells are converted into T-cells, B-cells and K-cells. Stem cells are transformed into T-cells in the thymus, the small organ just under the breastbone in children that begins to atrophy with age. Stem cells are converted into B-cells possibly in the bone marrow or a yet-to-be-located area equivalent to an organ in chickens called the *bursa of Fabricius.*

These specialized lymphocyte cells (B-, T- and K-cells) are stored in the lymphoid tissues such as the lymph nodes under the arms, behind the ear, in the groin and in other locations.

When an invader (antigen) is detected, the immune system responds by releasing one or more of its specialized lymphocytes. Released T-cells multiply and surround the invader. Once the invader has been isolated by rings of T-cells, it is chemically attacked by these defenders. The T-cells can also summon macrophages from the reticuloendothelial system to digest the invader.

The B-cells can also be released; they then produce antibodies (immunoglobulins) that stick to the invader, thereby increasing the likelihood of its ingestion by macrophages. Antibodies immunoglobulin M (I_gM) and immunoglobulin G (I_gG) circulate in the blood, while immunoglobulin A (I_gA) circulates in saliva and fluids that bathe mucous membranes. At least one other antibody, immunoglobulin E (I_gE) exists, but little is known about it.

Antibodies are tailor-made to specifically lock onto each of the millions of different microorganisms that may invade a person. Macrophages cleanse the blood and lymph of foreign particulate matter and also produce interferon, the body's anti-viral compounds. Dr. Norbert Roberts of the University of Rochester Medical School notes, "In addition, macrophages' production of interferon may be one mechanism of their extensive *anti-tumor* activity, since interferon can render macrophages tumorcidal and can inhibit the growth of tumor cells directly. Interferon has not only anti-viral activity, but it also has cell-growth inhibitory activity."[3]

REFERENCES

1. Richard A. Passwater, *Selenium as Food and Medicine,* (New Canaan, Conn.: Keats Publishing, Inc., 1980, 89–92).
2. *Time,* (March 1973), 19:67.
3. N. Roberts, *National Institutes of Health Records,* (March 4, 1980).

Vitamin C's Role in Preventing Cancer

These studies are representative of dozens culled from an extensive collection of tables prepared by the Life Sciences Research Office of the Federation of American Societies for Experimental Biology, under contract to the FDA. The studies clearly demonstrate that a greater intake of foods containing vitamin C can help prevent a variety of cancers.

In an extensive 1990 study of 10,000 women (4,437 women with breast cancer, 4,341 controls in the general population, and 1,754 hospital controls), dietary intake prior to the onset of cancer was analyzed. It was discovered that the intake of vitamin C had "the most consistent statistically significant inverse association with breast cancer risk" (Howe et al.). Both pre- and post-menopausal women were examined for this study, with the analyses done separately. Among women who regularly had a higher consumption of fruits and vegetables containing beta-carotene, fiber and carotenoids, there was also a lessened risk of breast cancer.

In South Carolina a long-term study was conducted from 1977 through 1981 of men, including 207 who had esophageal cancer and several hundred other control cases, all from the same eight coastal counties of the state. The controls were matched according to race, age, residence and year of death. Of the 422 controls, 157 were hospitalized at some point but did not have cancer, and there were 265 non-cancer-related deaths. After adjustment for smoking and alcohol consumption (the leading risk factors for esophageal cancer), men whose diets showed a regularly low amount of fruits (especially citrus fruits) and juice faced a "significantly increased" risk of esophageal cancer. Overall, low intakes of vitamin C and fiber were associated with an increased risk of esophageal cancer (Brown et al., 1988).

A 1988 study of four case-control regions in the U.S. (New Jersey; Atlanta, Georgia; Los Angeles, Santa Clara and San Mateo, California) examined 871 people with cancer of the mouth and pharynx and compared them to 979 controls who were matched for age, sex and race. They were interviewed extensively on their tobacco and alcohol use, normal diet as an adult, medical history and occupation. In men and women with a decreased risk of oral cancer, a higher intake of vitamin C was found and protective effects were seen for fruit consumption. When derived from fruit, there was "a significant protective effect of vitamin C, vitamin A and fiber," McLaughlin et al. noted. Interestingly, this study was not designed specifically to address the influence of vitamin C, yet there it was, an important factor in lowering disease risk.

In France, 743 cases of esophageal cancer and 1,975 controls from the same region were compared by food and alcohol intake and tobacco use. It was found that those who had cancer regularly consumed less vitamin C and E than the controls, and a higher intake of sugars. A higher intake of butter was associated with a higher risk of esophageal cancer. Higher intakes of vitamin C and vitamin E were related to a descreased risk of esophageal cancer. "Higher intakes of several other vitamins (retinol, beta-carotene, niacin) also associated with significantly decreased risk" of cancer, Tuyns et al. reported in 1987.

You would expect a study of lung-cancer patients to include a vast majority of smokers, but this particular research, conducted on women in Hong Kong, contained no one with a known history of smoking. The 88 cases of lung cancer were compared with

137 controls, all from the same districts. All of the subjects were interviewed as to regularly eaten foods, and the women with cancer gave their typical intake up to one-year prior to their diagnosis. A high consumption of leafy greens, carrots, tofu, fresh furit and fresh fish were found to have a "protective effect" against adenocarcinoma and large cell cancer. Eating lots of fresh fruits was found to offer protection against squamous cell tumors. Based on these results, the researchers (Koo et al., 1988) concluded that vitamin C, retinol and calcium (known to be in these foods) help protect against certain cancers.

A case-controlled study in China reported in 1988 showed that an increased consumption of vitamin C, calcium and carotene—all associated with high intakes of fresh fruit and vegetables—had a clearly protective effect against gastric cancer. Scientists compared 564 patients with stomach cancer to 1,131 population-based controls that were matched for age and sex. Besides interviewing research subjects on their medical history, occupation and smoking history, researchers had them answer an 85-item food-frequency questionnaire. Those who had a diet high in fruit and vegetables showed a decline in risk of gastric cancer (You et al.).

New Yorkers who eat more calories, fat, carbohydrates and iron than others of the same sex, race, age and neighborhood face a higher risk of contracting rectal cancer, a case-controlled study showed. When 422 patients with rectal cancer were compared with 422 of their peers, it was found that those who had higher intakes of carotenoids, vitamin C and vegetable fiber had a decreased risk of contracting the disease. This study by Freudenheim et al. was done in 1990 and judged to be a "well-conceived study" by peers in the research field.

Another New York study examined 428 cases of colon cancer, which were compared to 428 individual controls matched for age, sex and neighborhood. In the extensive interview about food intake (which was similar to that used in the Freudenheim research mentioned above) a number of factors emerged as important risk indicators. The risk of colon cancer was "positively associated with increasing intake of total fats" (predominantly animal fats) and total calories. On the other hand, there was "significantly reduced risk" of colon cancer associated with high intakes of tomatoes, peppers, carrots, onions and celery (Graham et al., 1988).

Cervical cancer risk is another type that can apparently be reduced with regular intake of vitamin C from vegetables and fruit. According to a case-controlled study of 189 cases of cervical cancer and 227 matched controls done in Washington state, a decreased risk was associated with high intakes of vitamin C. Increased intakes of dark green or yellow vegetables and fruit juices were associated with "significantly reduced" risk of cervical cancer (Verreault et al., 1989).

In a post-mortem study of 102 cancer deaths over a two-year period in Basel, Switzerland, it was discovered that the presence of vitamin C in the blood (after adjustment for smoking, which affects vitamin C levels and usage in the body) was significantly lower among those who died from stomach cancer.

APPENDIX C

Vitamin E's Action in Preventing Cancer

These studies are representative of dozens culled from an extensive collection of tables prepared by the Life Sciences Research Office of the Federation of American Societies for Experimental Biology, under contract to the FDA. The studies clearly demonstrate that a greater intake of foods containing vitamin E can help prevent a variety of cancers.

In the Netherlands in 1989 a study of 71 cases of people with squamous cell cancer of the head and neck with only one tumor and 17 cases of the same cancer who had at least two tumors included measurements of the serum levels of vitamins A, E and beta-carotene. Although no difference was found between the two groups in beta-carotene levels, there were "statistically significant differences" between the groups for serum vitamin A and vitamin E levels. According to de Vries et al. in this study, those with only one tumor had higher levels of A and E than those with two or more tumors.

A case-controlled study of four regions of the U.S. (New Jersey, Atlanta, and three cities in California including Los Angeles) 190 cases of oral and pharyngeal cancers were compared with 201 population-based controls matched for age and sex. All of the subjects were African-Americans. After accounting for alcohol and tobacco use, as well as food intake, occupation and medical history, it was found that there was a decreased risk of oral and pharyngeal cancers in men with higher levels of carotene and vitamin E. Also, the greater the intake of fruits and vegetables, the lower the risk of oral cancer in men and women (although the protection effect was stronger for men). There was a similar decline in risk associated with intake of vitamin C and fiber, Gridley et al. found in 1990.

A significant association between vitamin E intake and relative risk of esophageal cancer was seen in a French research study of 743 cases of men and women with esophageal cancer and 1,975 controls from the same region. Higher intakes of E were "associated with significantly decreased risk" of this cancer. Patients with cancer were also found to consume more sugars and starches than the control group, with an increased risk seen in those who consumed more butter. (Tuyns et al., 1987)

In a cross-sectional study of South Africans and esophageal cancer, van Helden et al. found that levels of vitamins A and E and red-cell levels of folate were significantly different. For each nutrient, the highest concentrations were found in the low-risk group. All concentrations, however, were within the lower range of clinically acceptable levels for these nutrients, the scientists noted. This was especially true for vitamin E, according to the 1987 research.

A randomized, double-blind, placebo-controlled crossover design research experiment was conducted in South Africa on 105 women with mammographic evidence of benign breast disease. Over 31 percent of the women had benign tumors, almost 24 percent had ductal hyperplasia, while 19 percent had benign tumors and fibroadenosis, and fibrocystic disease was present in 16 percent. After menstrual, dietary, reproductive, smoking and family health histories were collected, the cases were given 600 mg of alpha-tocopherol or a placebo for three months. Then they returned for another exam and the supplements were switched. Of the 83 cases who completed this trial, 37 percent of the women experienced improvement while on the vitamin E; 19 on the placebo. In the vitamin E group 16 cases of benign breast disease showed improvements that were evident on the follow-up mammograms (Meyer et al., 1990). Unfortunately, due to the relatively small size of this study, these results are not considered "statistically significant." However, they certainly indicate the need for larger studies into the positive effects of vitamin E on various conditions of cystic breasts.

In a case-control study of 69 cancer deaths in the Netherlands reported in 1987, baseline blood samples were analyzed for serum a-tocopherol, beta-carotene, retinol, selenium and cholesterol. Vitamin E levels were "inversely associated with risk of all cancers." Furthermore, among the 18 cases of lung cancer, there was a 9 percent lower level of the vitamin present than in the matched control subjects. (Kok et al., 1987)

Over 1,000 gastric cancer patients were studied and compared with age- and sex-matched controls from the same area of Italy. The results of extensive examination of smoking, occupational, medical, family and dietary history revealed that there was a lower risk of gastric cancer among subjects who regularly consumed nutrients including vitamins C, E and beta-carotene. The greater the intake of C and E, the lower the risk of stomach cancer. (Much of the vitamin intake was believed to be associated with the amount of olive oil used.) Increased risk of cancer was also associated with increasing intakes of protein and nitrites. (Buiatti et al., 1990)

Cancer of the pancreas is a notoriously deadly form of this disease. But in a case-controlled study in Maryland, among groups of 44 controls and 22 cases of pancreatic cancer matched for various factors, blood samples showed a protective effect of even low levels of vitamin E. (Burney et al., 1989)

A case-control study in France of 208 subjects included 70 people with digestive cancer, 34 people with colonic polyps, and 78 healthy controls. Blood samples were taken from all; the samples from the subjects with cancer and polyps were taken before any radiation, surgery or chemotherapy was performed. The amounts of retinol and vitamin E were found to be significantly lower in the subjects with digestive cancer than in the controls. There were no differences between the polyp group and the controls, according to Charpiot et al., as published in 1989.

Thirty cases of cervical intraepithelial neoplasia were studied and compared to 45 controls in a 1990 study in London. Serum samples were analyzed for vitamins E and A. The mean levels of serum vitamin E showed a "significant decreasing trend lower" in the cases versus the controls. Higher levels of vitamin E in the blood were shown to be protective against this condition, and this trend was even clearer when adjustments were made among the subjects for sexual history, smoking, and oral contraceptive use. (Cuzick et al., 1990)

Another significant study also showed the protective effects of vitamins E and A in a daily diet against cervical cancer, when compared with cases of others with abnormal cytology (without cancer) and a set of controls. Palan et al. performed a cross-sectional study of women in New York City in 1991, in which blood samples were collected prior to any treatment for cancer. In all of the cases of dysplasia and cervical cancer, "mean levels of vitamins A and E were significantly reduced." Also, there was an inverse association between the levels of nutrients and the severity of the cervical dysplasia.

A case-control study done in Washington state by Verreault et al. in 1989 showed that high vitamin E intake was significantly associated with a lower risk of cervical cancer. The subjects, which included 189 women with cervical cancer and 227 randomly selected controls, were extensively interviewed on their health and reproductive history, smoking, height and weight, whether they took vitamin supplements, use of contraceptives and age at first intercourse, number of sex partners, and history of cervical or vaginal infections. Subjects with higher dietary intakes of vitamin E showed lower risk. Supplement use of vitamins E and A was also associated with lesser risk of cervical cancer, as was more frequent consumption of dark green or yellow vegetables and fruit juices.

The amount of vitamin C consumed was also inversely related to risk of cancer, researchers noted.

Even deadly skin cancer has been shown to be affected by dietary intake of vitamin E. When Stryker et al. did a case-control study in Boston of 204 cases of malignant melanoma and compared them with 248 control patients, higher levels of E were associated with a decreased risk of the disease. Intake of vitamin E from food alone was also significantly associated with decreased risk of cancer, with subjects who consumed higher levels of E showing a proportionately lowered risk. The researchers examined the subjects' cooking habits (particularly use of fats), supplement intake, skin pigment characteristics, medical history and lifestyle factors in this definitive 1990 study.

A 1991 study of blood samples from 436 patients with a variety of cancers and 765 matched control subjects in Maryland was unusual in that no dietary history or notes about supplement use were included. But when the serum vitamin E levels were tallied, the odds ratios for four different cell types of lung cancer were all increased in cases of low serum E. A definite dose-responsive trend toward protection against lung cancer was noted with higher levels of vitamin E. And serum vitamin E levels were lower in cases of rectum, lung, prostate, bladder and colon cancer as well, than in the control group. (Comstock et al., 1991)

Gey et al. in Switzerland followed 3,000 initially healthy men over a period of seven years. During this time, there were 268 deaths which included 102 (38 percent) due to cancer. Blood samples conducted periodically throughout the study showed there were significantly lower levels of vitamin E present in the cancer group as a whole when compared with the 2,707 controls (survivors). Among those who died from gastrointestinal cancer, there were found to be significantly lower levels of vitamin E in the samples. Final trend analysis as reported in 1987 demonstrated that lower levels of vitamins E, A and beta-carotene "were associated with increased risk of death from all cancer."

The Influence of Vitamin A and Carotenoids on Cancer

These studies were culled from an extensive collection of tables prepared by the Life Sciences Research Office of the Federation of American Societies for Experimental Biology, under contract to the FDA. They demonstrate a clear association between the presence of vitamin A and carotenoids and a reduced risk of cancer.

A case-control study in Hong Kong compared 88 cases of women (without a history of smoking) who had lung cancer with 137 matched control subjects from the same area. A significantly increased risk of lung cancer was found to be associated with low intakes of fresh fruit and fish. A protective effect of a diet high in leafy green vegetables, carrots, tofu, fresh fruit and fresh fish was seen. Fresh fruits were also linked with protection against squamous cell tumors. (Koo et al., 1988)

When 64 patients with lung cancer were compared to 63 control subjects, all males, blood levels of beta-carotene and vitamin A were found to be significantly lower among the cancer cases, according to this research from Melbourne, Australia by Kune et al. in 1989.

The vitamins A, C, and fiber from fruit sources were found to have a protective effect against oral and pharyngeal cancer in an extensive case-controlled study covering four regions of the U.S.: New Jersey, Atlanta, two cities in Southern California and San Mateo. Normal dietary intake as an adult was examined, as well as tobacco and alcohol use, medical history, occupation and demographics in 871 patients with cancer and 979 population-based controls who were matched for age, race and sex. The results showed the protective effects of fruit consumption, with those in the top fourth group in terms of fruit intake having only half the risk of cancer as the group who ate the least amount of fruit. (McLaughlin et al., 1988)

An extensive French study compared 743 cases of esophageal cancer with 1,975 controls from the same area. Responses to a food-frequency questionnaire showed that those who had more niacin, retinol and beta-carotene in their diet had a "significantly decreased risk" of esophageal cancer. The risk also decreased when larger amounts of vitamin C-rich foods were included in the diet. Vitamin E intake and lessened risk also were associated, according to Tuyns et al. in 1987.

Beta-carotene was shown to have a significantly protective effect against colon cancer according to a case-control study done in Utah and reported in 1989. There were 231 newly-diagnosed cases of cancer compared to 391 cancer-free subjects in this study, which examined health history, height and weight, physical activity and dietary data (in the form of a 99-item food-frequency questionnaire) among all subjects. Beta-carotene intake was related to a lessened risk of colon cancer among male and female subjects; fiber proved protective in women; and cruciferous vegetables lessened the risk of colon cancer for men. (West et al., 1989)

A strictly dietary analysis of 4,437 cases of women with breast cancer versus 4,341 population controls and 1,754 hospital control subjects was done by Howe et al. and reported in 1990. Vitamin C had "the most consistent statistically significant inverse association" with risk of breast cancer. There was also a significantly lessened risk of the disease associated with total vitamin A, C, beta-

carotene and fiber intake. The risk of breast cancer in postmenopausal women was higher among those who had a higher intake
of saturated fats.

A small cross-sectional study of women in New York City who
had a variety of cancers was performed. Researchers examined the
levels of nutrients in the normal, benign and malignant tissues of
the cancer patients, and compared them with samples of normal
tissue from the same subjects for beta-carotene content. The concentrations of beta-carotene were found to be lower in all the
cancerous tissues when compared to adjacent "normal" tissue.
(Palan et al., 1989)

Another New York City study by Palan et al. done in 1988 compared over 100 women with cervical cancer, abnormal pap smears,
mild and severe dysplasia, to 37 control subjects. Blood sample
comparisons showed that mean plasma concentrations of beta-
carotene were significantly lower in all cases of dysplasia and cancer
when compared to the normal group. Those with cancer had the
lowest levels of beta-carotene; the women with severe dysplasia
had the next lowest, and those with mild dysplasia showed slightly
higher levels of beta-carotene than the former.

A 1988 study of Japanese men with prostate cancer and those
without compared occupation, medical and sexual history, and dietary intake. Low intakes of vitamin A (in the form of retinol
and beta-carotene) were associated with increased risk of cancer,
according to Ohno et al. and Oishi et al. Vitamin A and beta-
carotene from green and yellow vegetables was found to be significantly protective, the researchers noted. Interestingly, the risk
reduction associated with beta-carotene and A was seen in men
age 70 and older, but not younger (50–69).

Stahelin et al. of Basel, Switzerland published the results of their
comprehensive study of almost 3,000 people in 1987. This prospective cohort study examined blood samples from 2,974 people
over two years. Among this group there were 204 deaths from

cancer. Compared to the survivors, those who died from cancer had "significantly lower plasma carotene levels;" vitamin C was also lower in all cancer cases than in the surviving controls. Carotene levels were found to be significantly lower in the victims of stomach and lung cancers. Low carotene levels were also associated with an increased risk for lung cancer after adjustments were made for smoking, cholesterol levels and age. And, among all cancers, the combination of low levels of vitamin A and beta-carotene was associated with increased risk of the disease.

APPENDIX E

Dietary Fiber and Cancer Prevention

These studies are representative of dozens culled from an extensive collection of tables prepared by the Life Sciences Research Office of the Federation of American Societies for Experimental Biology, under contract to the FDA. The studies clearly demonstrate that a higher intake of dietary fiber can help prevent colorectal cancers.

In one study comparing colorectal cancer markers and fiber (Alberts et al., 1990), 17 patients ages 54 to 70 were selected to participate because of their high risk of recurrent colorectal cancer. Besides their usual diet, they took at least 13 grams of fiber in the form of All-Bran wheat-based supplement a day. After eight weeks of fiber supplementation, rectal biopsies showed an overall lower proliferation of cancerous cells: 22 percent lower. Assessments of this study determined that the results appeared to confirm the beneficial action of the addition of wheat bran fiber to the diet in these patients.

Another, much longer-term study by Freudenheim et al. reported in 1990 also showed that increased intakes of vitamin C, carotenoids and vegetable fiber were protective against rectal cancer. Lasting from 1978 to 1986, this study examined 277 men with cancer and 145 women with cancer, and compared them to equal-sized control groups (without cancer).

From January 1986 through March 1988 a population-based, case-referenced study was conducted on diet, body mass and colorectal cancer. Over 700 cancer patients and about 600 controls answered food-frequency questionnaires that were analyzed for fiber content. The colon and rectal cancer patients had followed their usual diet for at least five years before receiving the diagnosis of cancer. The carefully conducted study showed that the relative risk of colon and rectal cancer was decreased when a high-fiber diet was routinely eaten (Gerhardsson de Verdier, 1990).

Another study of almost 89,000 women ranging in age from 34 to 59 followed them during the years from 1980 through 1986. Using dietary questionnaires and estimations of fiber content in their diets, researchers examined the relationships between the intakes of meat, fat and fiber and colon cancer. As of 1986, there were 150 incidents of colon cancer. The scientists determined that a low intake of fiber from fruits *was* associated with increased risk of colon cancer, but that this was not statistically independent of meat intake (Willett et al., 1990).

Besides colorectal cancer, associations have been found between low-fiber diets and an increased risk of breast cancer. One population-based, case-controlled study conducted from 1985 through 1987 compared the intake of dietary fiber and beta-carotene with breast cancer risk. There were 133 cases of cancer among women 25 to 44 years old, compared to a control group of 238 women ages 55 to 64. Their dietary intake was estimated from interviews, so there was some uncertainty of the actual dietary intakes. However, fiber intake in the form of cereal products was found to be lower among the women with cancer than the control group. The amount of beta-carotene ingested seemed to be about the same for both. However, the results suggested that a diet rich in vegetable products may help lower the risk of breast cancer (Van't Veer et al., 1990).

APPENDIX F

Dietary Fat Intake and Risk of Cancer

These studies examining the relationship between dietary fat and various types of cancer are excerpted from the list of tables prepared by the Life Sciences Research Office of the Federation of American Societies for Experimental Biology, under contract to the FDA. The research studies that follow are by no means exhaustive, nor are they meant to be. They have been selected as highlights because they are representative of the information that the government and the scientific community in the U.S. have.

A case-control study of breast cancer patients in Quebec examined the menstrual, drug and tobacco, diet and physical activity histories of 290 newly diagnosed women as compared to 645 age-matched controls without cancer. Increased intake of carotenoid and fiber was associated with a decrease in high-risk features as shown on mammograms. (The relationship of mammographic indicators to dietary and fat factors and breast cancer risk was assessed in the controls only.) An increase in saturated fat intake was associated with an increase in high-risk factors, according to Brisson et al. in 1989.

Within a year of their diagnosis of breast cancer, 1,474 cases of breast cancer answered a lengthy questionnaire about their food intake; supplement use; and use of caffeinated beverages, sugar and artificial sweeteners. These patients' questionnaires were then compared with those of 1,322 age-stratified, randomly selected controls. "There was a significant trend for increased risk with increased intake of total fat," researchers Ewertz and Gill reported in 1990. These findings remained unchanged after the subjects' menstrual and reproductive histories were factored in to the study. The year delay in food-intake questioning among the women with breast cancer was to make sure no one was currently undergoing chemotherapy, which could radically change their diet and appetite.

Another case-control study in France examined 120 women with breast cancer and compared them to 109 controls. Nutritional habits, food frequency, reproductive and health histories were taken. Gerber et al. conducted this study over a four-year period and reported their results in 1989. They discovered that postmenopausal cases consumed more total fat and significantly more saturated and monounsaturated fats than postmenopausal controls. Plasma total cholesterol levels were also higher among the women with breast cancer. There was also evidence of lower lipid peroxidation in cases than in controls.

Yet another study corroborating the relationship between fat intake and breast cancer was reported by Holm et al. of Stockholm in 1989. Among 240 women of various ages with breast cancer, those with larger tumors were found to have consumed a higher percentage of calories as total fat and monounsaturated fat. They also had lower intakes of carbohydrates and fiber as a percentage of their total calories on a regular basis.

Subjects obtained from the National Health and Nutrition Examination Survey I Epidemiologic Follow-Up Study were compared to almost 200 women with breast cancer. The number of factors that were associated with increased risk of cancer included obesity and percentage of body fat, family history, age at first menarche, and fat intake. A "significant inverse association" was found between both total fat and saturated fat intake and risk of breast cancer, Jones et al. concluded in 1987.

In Singapore, 200 cases of breast cancer were compared to 420 hospital-based, age-matched control subjects by Lee et al. in 1991. Extensive histories that were taken and compared examined: menstrual and reproductive history, use of oral contraceptives, breast-feeding, tobacco use, family health history, height and weight, and education. The food frequency questionnaire featured 90 items and was used to assess intakes of animal and vegetable proteins, fat, saturated fatty acids, cholesterol, caffeine and certain nutrients. After the analyses were adjusted for age and other known risk factors, a significant increase in risk of cancer was found in pre-menopausal women with higher intakes of red meat and high proportions of total protein intake from animal sources. Significantly decreased risks were found, according to researchers, to be linked with the intake of beta-carotene, soy protein and total soy products consumed regularly, as well as with the intake of polyunsaturated fatty acids and the ratio of polyunsaturated acids to saturated fat intake.

In 1989 Toniolo et al. found in a case-control study in Italy that breast cancer cases consumed more animal protein and fat than the control group of women without cancer. Also, reduced risk was associated with decreased intakes of saturated fat and animal protein.

Breast cancer is by no means the only type of cancer affected by dietary fat intake. One study in Majorca, Spain, compared 286 people with colorectal cancer to 295 controls. Subjects were asked about their occupational, medical, pharmacological histories as well as any exposures to toxins. They also answered a 99-item food frequency questionnaire. An increased risk for colorectal cancer was seen among those with diets high in cereal (white bread and pasta). There was also a "significant trend for increased risk associated with education and weight," Benito et al. reported in 1990. Fresh meats (such as lamb and game) were associated with a higher risk for colon cancer, while an increased risk of rectal cancer was linked with a higher consumption of dairy products. A protective effect was seen for higher intakes of cruciferous vegetables overall. Furthermore, the researchers concluded, the combination of a high consumption of fresh meat, dairy products and refined cereals and starches, combined with a low intake of cruciferous vegetables, was associated with a four-fold increase in risk for colorectal cancer.

Freudenheim et al. conducted a case-controlled study in New York which was reported in 1990. They concluded, after comparing 422 people with rectal cancer to 422 sex-, age- and race-matched controls, that there was an increased risk of rectal cancer among those with an increased intake of calories, fat, carbohydrates and iron. Those with greater intakes of carotenoids, vitamin C, and dietary fiber from vegetable sources had a decreased risk of rectal cancer. The association between fat and risk was seen to be most significant among male subjects, the researchers noted, with a somewhat lesser association for women, in this "well-conceived study."

Higher intakes of dietary fat were also found to be related to incidences of colorectal cancer in Melbourne, Australia, according to Kune et al. in 1987. This case-control study of over 1,400 subjects concluded that there was a "dose-dependent inverse relationship between fiber, vitamin C, beta-carotene, total vegetables, and cruciferous vegetable" intake and cancer risk. Vitamin supplements were judged "highly protective," while high intakes of fat were a "contributing factor in the overall risk factor model, especially for men," the study reported.

A case-control study in Utah of 229 colon cancer cases and 384 randomly selected controls found that calories, protein and fat were all associated with an increased risk of colon cancer. Interestingly, the amount of total physical activity had a protective effect; an analysis of the data suggested that "physical activity modifies colon cancer risk associated with diet." Although exercise was protective in both men and women, "intense" physical activity was found to be most protective in men. The American way of life—and in particular, eating—is proving hazardous to the health of the Chinese and Chinese-Americans, according to a study published in 1990 by Whittemore et al., and conducted in the U.S. and China. Thousands of subjects were interviewed about their diet, physical activity, menstrual factors, demographic characteristics and patterns of residence. The dietary analysis was based on an 84-item food-frequency questionnaire. The interviews were based on the year prior to the diagnosis of colorectal cancer for these cases and the year before the interview for the cancer-free controls. Of the 905 cases of colorectal cancer, 473 of the patients were from North America and 432 were from China. There were 2,488 controls in this study (1,192 Chinese-Americans from North America, and 1,296 subjects from China). Most of the North American cancer cases and controls were born in Asia. The results showed that, among the Chinese-American participants, there was "significant risk associated with duration of residence in North America." Furthermore, the colorectal cancer patients "tended to be more Westernized" than the controls. In both continents, the ones with cancer had regularly consumed more calories, protein, fat and cholesterol than the cancer-free control group. "There was a significant protective effect of vegetable consumption among Chinese-American men and women and in Chinese men," the research showed. Sedentary lifestyle was also found to be a significant risk factor for cancer. Saturated fat in particular was strongly linked to risk of colorectal cancer, with this effect seen most strongly in the U.S. sample. This reflects the typical American diet which is heavy in meat and dairy products. Whittemore and colleagues concluded that a lack of physical activity and a diet high in saturated fat was estimated to account for 60 and 40 percent of colorectal cancer incidence among Chinese-American men and women, respectively.

When 150 cases of colon cancer in women were compared to 88,601 female controls from the Nurses Health Study, an increased risk of colon cancer was found to be related to the total fat, saturated and monounsaturated fats, and animal fats consumed. A higher intake of beef, pork or lamb as a main dish was highly related to cancer risk, as was the ratio intake of red meat to intake of chicken and fish. Eating fish and chicken without the skin offered some protection against colon cancer. (Willett et al., 1990)

In a case-control study in Louisiana of 363 cases of pancreatic cancer and 1,234 hospital-based, matched controls, data was obtained on smoking, occupational and residential history, alcohol use, family and medical health history, leisure activities, and diet. Here, where barbecue is king, it was found that risk of cancer of the pancreas was clearly associated with the intake of pork products (including bacon, ham, sausage, cold cuts and unprocessed fresh pork) and rice. In men, a higher intake of dairy products was also positively associated with increased risk. However, fresh fruit, juice and vitamin C were shown to have a protective effect against pancreatic cancer; in fact, "fruit also conferred a protective effect against intake of pork products," researchers Falk et al. reported in 1988.

A higher intake of beef and pork was linked to greater risk of death from pancreatic cancer in a study of 212 cancer deaths compared to 220 controls in Minnesota. A decreased risk of pancreatic cancer was associated with the intake of cruciferous vegetables. (Olsen et al., 1989)

In another study of this particularly deadly form of cancer, 110 cases were compared with 195 randomly selected controls matched for age, sex and region in southwestern Poland. There was a "significant trend towards increased risk associated with cholesterol intake," Zatonski et al. concluded in 1991, and "a significant inverse relationship between vitamin C intake and risk."

A case-control study of newly diagnosed prostate cancer cases in Japan examined marital, medical, occupational and religious histories; dietary intake; body type and sex life. When compared with a matched control group, low intakes of vitamin A (retinol and carotene) were associated with increased risk of cancer of the prostate. Vitamin A and beta-carotene from green and yellow vegetables were judged to be "significantly protective." (Ohno et al. and Oishi et al., 1988)

In Stockholm, Sweden, 418 subjects with urothelial cancer and/or squamous cell cancer of the lower urinary tract were compared to 511 age-matched controls. Based on health and medical histories and dietary intake, researchers determined that total fat and fried foods were "significantly associated with increased risk." Supplemental vitamin A was inversely associated with risk. (Steineck et al., 1990)

An international, cross-sectional study of people in 20 countries examined the average cancer incidence data for breast, cervix, prostate, colon and lung for the years 1973 through 1977. The estimates for the per capita food, fiber, fat and caloric intake were taken from the Food Balance Sheets published by the United Nations Food and Agricultural Organization. Total fat intake was strongly associated with cancer of the breast, colon and prostate, even after adjustment for total calorie intake. Saturated fat was positively associated with incidence of cancers of the breast, colon and prostate; poly-unsaturated fat was associated with incidence of breast and prostate cancers. Cancers of the lung and cervix were not correlated with dietary fat intake. Fiber intake affected the magnitude of the fat cancer correlations, especially between total fat and colon cancer. (Hursting et al., 1990)

BIBLIOGRAPHY AND ADDITIONAL READING

Anderson, Robert A. *Wellness Medicine*. New Canaan, Connecticut: Keats Publishing, Inc., 1987.

Bland, Jeffrey, editor. *Medical Applications of Clinical Nutrition*. New Canaan, Connecticut: Keats Publishing, Inc., 1983.

Braverman, Eric R. and Pfeiffer, Carl C. *The Healing Nutrients Within*. New Canaan, Connecticut: Keats Publishing, Inc., 1987.

Cameron, Ewan and Pauling, Linus. *Cancer and Vitamin C*. Menlo Park, California: Linus Pauling Institute of Science and Medicine, 1979.

Cameron, Ewan. *Hyaluronidase and Cancer*. Elmsford, New York: Pergamon Press, 1966.

Clark, Linda. *Know Your Nutrition*. New Canaan, Connecticut: Keats Publishing, Inc., 1973.

Colgan, Michael. *Prevent Cancer Now*. San Diego, California: C. I. Publications, 1990.

Committee on Diet, Nutrition and Cancer. *Diet, Nutrition and Cancer: Directions for Research*. Washington, D.C.: National Academy Press, 1983.

Culbert, Michael L. *Freedom from Cancer*. New York: Pocket Books, 1977.

Fink, John M. *Third Opinion: An International Directory to Alternative Therapy Centers for the Treatment and Prevention of Cancer*. Garden City, New York: Avery Publishing Group, Inc., 1988.

Fredericks, Carlton. *Breast Cancer: A Nutritional Approach*. New York: Grossett & Dunlap, Inc., 1977.

213

Garrison, Robert H. and Somer, Elizabeth. *The Nutrition Desk Reference*. New Canaan, Connecticut: Keats Publishing, Inc., 1990.

Goodman, Sandra. *Vitamin C: The Master Nutrient*. New Canaan, Connecticut: Keats Publishing, Inc., 1991.

Greenberg, Kurt, editor. *Challenging Orthodoxy*. New Canaan, Connecticut: Keats Publishing, Inc., 1991.

Heinerman, John. *The Treatment of Cancer with Herbs*. Orem, Utah: BiWorld Publishers, 1984.

Hoffer, Abram. *Orthomolecular Medicine for Physicians*. New Canaan, Connecticut: Keats Publishing, Inc., 1989.

Hoffer, Abram and Walker, Morton. *Orthomolecular Nutrition*. New Canaan, Connecticut: Keats Publishing, 1978.

Hsu, Hong-yen. *Treating Cancer with Chinese Herbs*. Long Beach, California: Oriental Healing Arts Institute, 1990.

Kittler, Glenn D. *Laetrile—Control for Cancer*. New York: Warner Paperback, 1963.

Kugler, Hans. *Seven Keys to a Longer Life*. New York: Stein and Day, 1978.

Lane, William I. and Comac, Linda. *Sharks Don't Get Cancer*. Garden City, New York: Avery Publishing Group, Inc., 1992.

Lien, Eric J. and Li, Wen Y. *Anti-Cancer Chinese Drugs*. Long Beach, California: Oriental Healing Arts Institute, 1985.

Mervyn, Len. *Minerals and Your Health*. New Canaan, Connecticut: Keats Publishing, Inc., 1984.

Moss, Ralph W. *Cancer Therapy*. New York: Equinox Press, 1992.

Moss, Ralph W. *The Cancer Industry*. New York: Paragon House, 1989.

Mowrey, Daniel B. *Herbal Tonic Therapies*. New Canaan, Connecticut: Keats Publishing, Inc., 1993.

Oden, Clifford. *Thank God I Have Cancer!* Los Altos, California: Choice Publications, 1977.

Passwater, Richard A. *Selenium as Food and Medicine*. New Canaan, Connecticut: Keats Publishing, Inc., 1980.

Passwater, Richard A. *Selenium Update*. New Canaan, Connecticut: Keats Publishing, Inc., 1987.

Passwater, Richard A. *The New Supernutrition*. New York: Pocket Books, 1991.

Passwater, Richard A. and Cranton, Elmer M. *Trace Elements, Hair Analysis and Nutrition.* New Canaan, Connecticut: Keats Publishing, Inc., 1983.

Pauling, Linus. *Vitamin C and the Common Cold.* San Francisco: W. H. Freeman, 1970.

Pfeiffer, Carl C. *Mental and Elemental Nutrients.* New Canaan, Connecticut: Keats Publishing, Inc., 1975.

Shute, Evan V. *The Heart and Vitamin E.* New Canaan, Connecticut: Keats Publishing, Inc., 1977.

Shute, Wilfrid E. *The Complete, Updated Vitamin E Book.* New Canaan, Connecticut: Keats Publishing, Inc., 1975.

Simone, Charles B. *Cancer & Nutrition, A 10-Point Plan to Reduce Your Chances of Getting Cancer.* New York: McGraw-Hill Book Company, 1992.

Stone, Irwin. *The Healing Factor: Vitamin C Against Disease.* New York: Grosset & Dunlap, 1972.

U.S. Department of Health & Human Services. *Diet, Nutrition & Cancer Prevention.* Bethesda, Maryland: National Institutes of Health Publication, 1984.

Werbach, Melvyn R. *Nutritional Influences on Illness.* New Canaan, Connecticut: Keats Publishing, Inc., 1988.

Williams, Roger J. and Kalita, Dwight K., editors. *A Physician's Handbook on Orthomolecular Medicine.* New Canaan, Connecticut: Keats Publishing, Inc., 1977.

Wright, Jonathan V. *Dr. Wright's Guide to Healing with Nutrition.* New Canaan, Connecticut: Keats Publishing, Inc., 1990.

INDEX

acidophilus bacteria, 156
Adamson, Dr. Richard, 11
adenocarcinoma, 27
Adriamycin (chemotherapy drug), 56
air pollution and cancer, 81
alcohol, a cancer promoter, 19, 26
  breast cancer risk and, 142–145
  colon cancer and, 162
  prostate cancer and, 173
  suppresses immune system, 26
alphacarotene, 34
AMC Cancer Research Center, 146
American Cancer Society, 11, 15, 40,
  112
American Health Foundation, 141, 174
American Hospital Association, 14
American Laboratory, 10
amygdalin, B-17: *see* laetrile
androgens and prostate cancer, 176
angiogenesis, 97
antineoplastons, 113
antioxidant nutrients, 18, 72–74
  aging and, 9
  beta-carotene, 32
  cancer prevention and 18, 53
  cervical cancer and, 182
  coenzyme Q-10 and, 32
  colon cancer and, 160
  free radicals and, 9, 10
  glutathione peroxidase and, 32
  hydroperoxidases and, 32
  immune system and, 9–10
  selenium and, 32
  skin cancer and, 168
  superoxide dismutase (SOD) and, 32

  thiol enzymes and, 32
  vitamin A and, 31
  vitamin C and, 31, 44
  vitamin E and, 32, 45
Arlin J. Brown Cancer Information
  Center, 121
ascorbate: *see* vitamin C
ascorbic acid: *see* vitamin C

B complex vitamins: *see* vitamin B
Bailar, Dr. John, 14
Bailey, Herb, 118
beer and colon cancer, 162
Beker, Dr. Dubrava, 147
Bendich, Dr. Adrienne, 54
benign breast disease, 134–135
benign prostatic hypertrophy (BPH),
  172
beta-carotene, 32, 33–41
  recommended daily consumption,
  34
  protects against certain cancers,
  38–39, 52
  strengthens immune function, 34
  vitamin E deficiency and, 52–53
  see also: antioxidants
BGC, 120
Bifidobacterium, 156
bile, 156–157
bioflavonoids, 91
birth control pills: *see* oral
  contraceptives
Bjelke, Dr. E., 36
bladder cancer, cause of, 20

217

ABOUT THE AUTHOR

More than 35 years of biochemical and nutritional experience go into this completely rewritten update of the book *Cancer and Its Nutritional Therapies*.

Richard Passwater's discoveries have led to worldwide recognition. He is listed in *Who's Who in the World, Who's Who in America, American Men and Women of Science,* and *Who's Who in the Frontiers of Science*. Yet he considers his greatest honors his family, his selection as "Citizen of the Year" in his community, the privilege of being the Chief of his Community's Volunteer Fire Department, and receiving the Nutrition Industry's Achievement Award in 1989.

Richard Passwater is a biochemist widely recognized for his health research. His laboratory experience in gerontology, nutrition, and spectroscopy has brought together diverse disciplines resulting in many discoveries, some of which have been patented in more than ten countries.

He is recognized as a leader in free-radical pathology and fluorometry, and a foremost expert in trace nutrients in health. He is a student of the scientific literature, as well as a laboratory experimenter.

The author is the Director of Research at the Solgar Nutritional Research Center in Ocean Pines, Berlin, Maryland, a division of Solgar Co., Inc., of Lynbrook, New York, in which he is also a corporate vice president.

He is currently a liaison to Congress for the American Chemical Society's Department of Government Relations and Science Policy.

The author has published several dozens of articles in the scientific literature on the aging process, cancer, cholesterol, selenium, dieting, and fluorometry.

His research emphases are in trace nutients having antioxidant capability and in isolating unidentified nutrients present in several natural foods but missing in refined synthetic diets containing all the "known" nutrients.

Previously, he has been Vice President of Research for the American Gerontological Research Laboratories, Inc., a division of Life Science Labs, Inc.; Applications Research Laboratory Director for the American Instrument division of Baxter-Travenol Laboratories, Inc.; and Supervisor of the Instrumental Analyses Laboratory for the Baker and Adamson division of Allied Chemical Corp., Inc.

The author's education includes a B.S. in Chemistry from the University of Delaware in 1959 and a Ph.D. in Biochemistry from Bernadean University in 1976.

He was certified by the American Chemical Society on August 27, 1959 and is a fellow status in the American Institute of Chemists.

The author is past Vice President of the International Foundation for Preventive Medicine, Inc. (1977–81), past-President of the American Academy of Applied Health Sciences (1982–84) and past-President of Sub-Aqueous Exploration, Inc. (1983–84). He was the Washington Representative for the Institute of Nutritional Research (1975–79), and a lecturer for the Donsbach University Outreach Program from 1978 through 1984.

Richard Passwater is a contributing editor for the *Journal of Applied Nutrition,* and serves on the editorial boards of *Whole Foods* and *VIM Newsletter.* He is a health columnist for *Whole Foods* and a past columnist for *Your Good Health.* In the past, he has been editor of *Fluorescence News,* on the editorial board of *Analytical Letters,* and a reviewer for *Analytical Chemistry.* He has served on the editorial boards of the *Journal of Holistic Medicine,* the official journal of the American Holistic Medical Association, and *Nutritional Perspectives.*

The author holds several international patents on formulations to prevent and treat cancer, and one on formulations for life extension. These patents, based on antioxidant nutrients, were filed starting in 1970 and today are the subject of research by the National Cancer Institute and other agencies. Human clinical trials confirming important parts of Richard Passwater's early animal studies have recently been published.[1, 2, 3]

Besides his discoveries in cancer and aging research, the author has contributed new concepts to nutritional science including the Supernutrition Principle of optimal nourishment, and the FLAB Concept of using FLAB Units and the FLAB index to better measure the effects of food on body chemistry. Current research by others confirms the FLAB Units and Index principles that different foods produce insulin responses quite different from those predicted by the previous teachings merely utilizing food composition tables in regard to carbohydrate type, protein and fat content.[4]

Other important research projects include a joint five-year study with Dr. Linus Pauling (Linus Pauling Institute) and Dr. James Enstrom (UCLA School of Public Health) of the benefits of vitamin supplements on a large group of Californian volunteers, and a study of the protective effect of vitamin E against heart disease. The Enstrom–Pauling study showed that the supplemented volunteers had only two-thirds the death rate expected for typical Californians of the same age, sex, race, etc.[5] [Proc. Natl. Acad. Sci. 79, 6023-7 (1982)] The vitamin E study was a retrospective study of vitamin E users which showed that long-term vitamin E users had less than half of the heart disease rate of typical Americans of the same age, sex, and race.[6] (Prevention, Jan.-Aug. 1978). The results of this study were confirmed in 1992 by two independent Harvard studies.

The author has been twice honored by the Committee For World Health for "Outstanding Research" (1978 and 1980). In 1976, he was a recipient of one of the Notable Americans awards. In 1973, he was a nominee for the American Chemical Society's Award in Chemical Education. In 1987, he received the "Citizen of the Year" Award in his hometown of Ocean Pines, Maryland, for his community service. In 1989 he was awarded the Nutrition Industry's Achievement Award by *Whole Foods* magazine.

One of his books was chosen by *Library Journal* as one of the top six health books for 1983, and one of the top 100 science and technology books in a field of 40,000 books. (*Trace Elements, Hair Analysis and Nutrition* with Dr. E. Cranton, Keats Publishing, Inc., New Canaan, Connecticut.)

He has authored several best-selling books which include *The New Supernutrition* (Pocket Books, 1991), *Trace Elements, Hair Analysis and Nutrition* with Elmer Cranton, M.D. (Keats Publishing, Inc. 1983), *Selenium as Food and Medicine* (Keats, 1980), *The Easy No-Flab Diet* (Marek, 1979), *Cancer and Its Nutritional Therapies* (Keats, 1978), *Super Calorie, Carbohydrate Counter* (Dale, 1978), and *Supernutrition for Healthy Hearts* (Pocket Books, 1976). The author is also the co-editor, with Dr. Earl Mindell, of a series of over 50 Good Health Guides from Keats Publishing, Inc., and has personally authored the following booklets: *Chromium Picolinate* (1992), *Pycnogenol* (1992, *Fish Oils Update* (1987), *Selenium Update* (1986), *Antioxidant Nutrients* (1985), *Beta-carotene* (1984), *Beginners' Vitamin Guide* (1983), *EPA-Marine Lipids* (1982), *GTF-Chromium* (1982) and *Evening Primrose Oil* (1981). His books have been translated into Spanish, French, Dutch, and Japanese.

The author's hobbies include photography, nature studies, wildlife art, genealogy, subaqueous exploration and archaeology.

REFERENCES

1. P. M. Horvath and C. Ip, "Synergistic effect of vitamine E and selenium in the chemoprevention of mammary carcinogenesis," *Cancer Research* (Nov. 1983) 43:5335–5341.
2. W. C. Willett et al., *Lancet* (July 1983) 130–4. "Prediagnostic serum selenium and risk of cancer."
3. N. J. Wald et al., "Plasma retinol, beta-carotene and vitamin E levels in relation to the future risk of breast cancer," *British Journal of Cancer* (1984) 49:321–4.
4. P. Capro, J. Olefsky, *New England Journal of Medicine* (July 7, 1983) 309(1):44–45.
5. Proc. National Academy of Science (1982) 79, 6023–7.
6. *Prevention* magazine, Jan. and Aug., 1978.